Rosemary Conley founded the SAGG Slimming and Good Grooming organization in 1972. Eight years later, after developing the business throughout Leicestershire, she sold it to IPC Magazines Ltd and was appointed Managing Director of Successful Slimming Clubs. Since 1986 she has taught her slimming philosophy on a freelance basis.

Rosemary Conley's Hip and Thigh Diet was developed, with medical advice, in an attempt to avoid surgery to remove her gall bladder. The book was published in 1988 and became an international number 1 bestseller. Together with the *Complete Hip and Thigh Diet*, published in 1989, it has sold over a million copies.

Rosemary, a born-again Christian, is married to Mike Rimmington, her partner in Rosemary Conley Enterprises. She has one daughter, Dawn, by her previous marriage. She lives in Leicester.

D1140165

Rosemary Conley's Guide to Fat in Food

GRAFTON BOOKS

A Division of the Collins Publishing Group

LONDON GLASGOW
TORONTO SYDNEY AUCKLAND

Grafton Books
A Division of the Collins Publishing Group
8 Grafton Street, London W1X 3LA

A Grafton Paperback Original 1989

A CIP catalogue record for this book
is available from the British Library

ISBN 0-586-20667-1

Printed and bound in Great Britain by
Cox and Wyman Ltd, Reading, Berks.

Set in Times

Contents

Introduction

'Plenty to eat' was the key to the success of my *Hip and Thigh Diet*, according to my diet trial team, followed by 'no calorie counting', 'freedom of choice of meals' and 'not having to weigh the food'. For the first time in dieting history, men and women all over the world found themselves *enjoying* losing weight. 'You can't call this a diet,' they said, 'it's more a "way of eating".' And it's all so incredibly simple. You just cut out altogether the very *high*-fat foods, choose in moderation foods *low* in fat, and eat liberal amounts of fruit and vegetables which are almost fat-free. By having three good low-fat meals a day, with no nibbling in between, we can re-educate our palate, improve our eating pattern, eat healthily *and* lose *weight and inches from all the right places*. And there's more – not only can we achieve a shape we never dreamed possible, we can actually *maintain* it too.

The failure rate of most other diets is disappointingly high. For the few who do succeed, their lack of long-term success is extremely disheartening.

This *Guide to Fat in Food* gives an at-a-glance view of the fat content in a vast variety of foods. The foods to be avoided almost shout at you, they're so full of fat. But the good news is the amazing number of foods containing little or no fat: foods which can be eaten liberally providing they are eaten at mealtimes.

'But what about calories? I thought you had to eat fewer calories than your body needs if you want to lose weight.'

This is true, of course, but when we realize that ounce for ounce fat contains twice as many calories as carbohydrate, it is plain to see we can eat *more food* yet *fewer calories*. Furthermore, doctors at the Harvard Medical School in the USA have researched the effects of high-fat calories compared with low-fat ones. The results showed that fatty foods laid down much more fat than non-fatty foods with the same calorie content. Providing you don't take carbohydrates in excess, after they have nourished you they will burn completely away. Fats, on the other hand, after fulfilling their energy-giving function, stay within the body and go to rest in those areas which are the first to *store* fat and the last to *reduce* by normal slimming methods. As soon as we reduce our fat intake *and* our calories, these fatty areas begin to burn up – thus the amazing inch losses experienced by those following my original *Hip and Thigh Diet* (Arrow, £2.99) and my *Complete Hip and Thigh Diet* (Arrow, £3.50).

'*So can you eat* more *calories if they're low-fat calories and still lose weight?*'

Yes – most certainly. Here is an example. On the left below is a typical calorie-counted diet menu amounting to approximately 1400 calories. On the right is a similar menu, typical of the *Hip and Thigh Diet*, offering approximately 1500 calories. All that has changed is the fat content of the menu.

Calorie-counted diet		*Low-fat diet*	
Breakfast			
Glass orange juice	50	Glass orange juice	50
1 boiled egg	90	1 slice toast	100
½ slice toast	50	(wholemeal bread)	
(wholemeal bread)		8 oz (200 g) baked beans	144
½ oz (12 g) low-fat spread	50		
Lunch			
Salad (mixed)	30	Large jacket potato	200
1½ oz (37 g) cheddar cheese	180	2 oz (50 g) chicken	100
Reduced-oil dressing	50	Salad (mixed)	30
Diet yogurt	50	2 oz (50 g) Branston pickle	90
Mid-afternoon			
1 Digestive biscuit	45		

Dinner

3 oz (75 g) beef	240	Melon wedge	20
3 oz (75 g) roast potatoes	150	8 oz (200 g) fish	160
2 oz (50 g) Yorkshire pudding	120	Unlimited vegetables	210
4 oz (100 g) peas	60	Tomato sauce	30
4 oz (100 g) carrots	20	2 pieces any fresh fruit	100
Gravy	50	2 glasses wine	200
½ pint (280 ml) milk	200	½ pint (280 ml) skimmed milk	100
Total calories	1435		1534

As you will see, there is vastly more to eat in the low-fat menu than in the calorie-counted one, and the slimmer could not possibly feel hungry. Both menus will effect a satisfactory weight loss, but, more significantly, the low-fat menu, despite its extra 100 calories, will work better in shifting actual fat (and inches) than the other one.

Having established that whilst calories *do* count, on the *Hip and Thigh Diet* they aren't quite so critical as in most diets, so we do not need to spend any more time discussing them. We know that there is more than enough good food we can eat, that there is no fear of becoming hungry, and that despite the higher intake of calories we *will* lose weight and inches. As one reader wrote: 'I'm writing to say thank you very much for bringing out a diet which doesn't really feel like one. I've been on lots of diets, usually calorie-counted ones, and get fed up and give up. I've been on yours for 5 weeks so far and I've lost about 12 lbs and I'm 8 stone 11 lbs which I haven't been for years. The menus I couldn't get over, they were so filling, and the ones for one person make two main meals for me, they are so generous.'

READ THIS BEFORE YOU USE THE TABLES
This is where the fat tables come in.

The line alongside each food represents the fat content in *one ounce* of that particular food. If we can learn which foods should always be avoided and which we can eat freely, our calorie- and unit-counting days can stay behind us for ever. It won't take long to memorize which cuts of meat contain least fat, which flavour of soup to choose, and that if you must have a biscuit a Jaffa Cake is better than a Digestive. Ryvita contains one sixth of the fat in a plain water biscuit – and did you know that sunflower margarines contain as much fat as ordinary butter? Or that French dressing is eighty per cent fat and therefore a disaster too?

Because I felt so strongly that a table in line-graph form was the clearest way to illustrate fat content, I had to make the decision to stick to a 25 g/1 oz measure. It is vital to consider what a normal *serving* might be. Multiply the fat content per ounce as shown in the book by however many ounces you are likely to eat and then judge whether it's acceptable or not.

For example, 1 ounce of frozen chips contains 5 grammes of fat compared with 1 ounce of crisps at 9 grammes. Whilst you might be happy with a small packet of crisps, you would hardly be satisfied if you only ate 2 ounces of chips containing a similar amount of fat. On the other hand, mustard and curry powder are quite high in fat but the amount you eat is minimal. If you ate a whole ounce of either you'd probably blow your head off. So it all must be taken in perspective.

This book will prove invaluable to anyone dining out, perhaps planning a dinner party menu or simply wishing to eat a low-fat diet for medical reasons. Whilst we have included many foods from major food manufacturers and retailers, there was little need to offer a more comprehensive guide as one brand does not usually vary very much from another. It is the average fat content that determines whether or not you decide to eat it. Thereafter, if you want, you can make a more detailed selection between brands. For instance, bread doesn't vary very much and is basically acceptable. Cakes, though, are to be discouraged, so a selection from Marks & Spencer, Sainsbury's, Waitrose and Tesco's really is more than sufficient to prove that most cakes contain a lot of fat.

If an item hasn't been included in this Guide, you can, of course, check on the packets and wrappers of products. The 'Nutrition' panel usually offers fat content per 100 grammes but sometimes per serving. Remember to make the necessary calculation. Divide the 100 gramme figure by 4 to give a comparable measure to those in this Guide.

It is almost impossible to list so many types of food under logical general headings – particularly when different names are given to various types of food depending on where you live! With this in mind we have tried to make the contents list on pages v–vi as informative as possible by cross-referencing some of the entries. So please read it carefully *before* consulting the fat tables themselves.

Certain products are so well known that they have become household names, and as such have been included under the 'General' heading in each section for easy reference.

Whilst every effort has been made to ensure the accuracy of these tables, it must be appreciated that alterations to ranges and recipes are constantly being made by manufacturers.

Obviously it is important that we eat a balanced diet. Again, if we can learn which foods make up our daily nutritional requirements our health and energy will benefit. We need different foods to fulfil a variety of functions: proteins for growth and repair, carbohydrates for energy, vitamins and minerals for general good health, and a minute amount of fat.

Each day try to include within your diet 6 oz (150 g) protein food (fish, poultry, meat, cottage cheese, baked beans, lentils and pulses); 6 oz (150 g) carbohydrate food (bread, cereals, potatoes, rice, pasta); 12 oz (300 g) vegetables (including salad); 12 oz (300 g) fresh fruit; 5 oz

(125 g) low-fat yogurt; ½ pt (280 ml) skimmed or semi-skimmed milk, or ordinary milk with the cream removed; and one multivitamin tablet. These daily nutritional requirements include an adequate supply of fat without the need to add any extra.

To sum up: if you are trying to lose weight and inches, avoid all foods which contain more than 2 grammes of fat per ounce, except those used in small quantities as flavourings or, for example, mustard, curry powder, or horse-radish.

After achieving your desired weight and shape, attempt to stick to foods still low in fat content without being too strict. If you dine out, relax and enjoy yourself. If it was a fairly high-fat meal, cut down the next day to counteract the damage.

'So if something contains no fat I can eat or drink it freely?'

No. Most alcohol, of course, contains no fat, but being high in calories – and harmful to health if taken in excess – it should be restricted to two drinks a day whilst on the diet. This can be increased for maintenance dieters, but women should remember that more than two drinks a day can be damaging to our health. Men are able to drink a little more without the same element of risk. Sugar is another thing to watch for. Sugar itself contains no fat, and being pure carbohydrate gives half the number of calories per ounce compared with fat, but those calories offer no nutrients, only energy. However, you are allowed to have some marmalade on your toast, honey on your porridge, sugar on your cereal, meringues (without cream of course), and fruit cooked or served in wine. Alcohol is, of course, another source of sugar. Anyone who never drinks alcohol may enjoy the occasional packet of lower-calorie sweets such as Polo mints or wine gums, but don't get into the bad habit of eating too many – remember they offer no nutrients, only empty calories.

'But don't we need a certain amount of fat?'

Almost all foods contain *some* fat. On a diet where you eat plenty of grains, vegetables and low-fat proteins, you will still be taking in more than adequate amounts of fat. Extensive investigations carried out in America have shown that as long as a diet provides adequate calories from a variety of foods we cannot be deficient in fat. Fat-deficient diets simply do not exist.

'But what about fats low in cholesterol and high in polyun-saturates? I thought they were good *for you.'*

I can understand anyone being confused by this argument. Because our bodies actually make an adequate supply of cholesterol, it *is* important for those with a history of heart disease to avoid foods high in cholesterol. Too much cholesterol can have the effect of accelerating the build-up of atheroma (furring up of the arteries) which in turn can lead to heart disease. However, taken in small quantities, fats, whether saturated or unsaturated, are unlikely to do actual harm to most people other than to make them fat. The difference between the two types is their chemical make-up, but their calorie content is equal. There are now some arguments *against* the use of unsaturated fats. Whilst both kinds of fats raise the triglyceride levels in the blood, there is evidence to indicate that after the consumption of unsaturated fat the level stays higher for longer. Also, it is suggested that polyunsaturates can deplete the body's level of vitamin E, a vitamin often recommended to women suffering from PMT. This would explain why many of my *Hip and Thigh* dieters – who were, of course, eating no obvious fats on the diet – experienced amazing relief of symptoms. By reducing our fat intake significantly, we maintain the body's natural balance of vitamin E. So cutting out all visible fats like butter, margarines (including those high in polyunsaturates) and vegetable oils is recommended for everyone, particularly those with a history of heart disease.

If you are a keen cook you will find this *Guide to Fat in Food* a great help in exchanging some ingredients for low-fat alternatives. Once you learn which foods are 'allowed' and which are unacceptable, you will be able to improvise to your heart's content and produce delicious meals that no one will believe are low-fat 'diet' menus. Exchange low-fat fromage frais or quark for soft cheeses, use yogurt instead of cream, and stir-fry in a non-stick pan, moistening only with water or stock as necessary.

Anyone following a low-fat diet would find these foods a good basis to have in their store cupboard: skimmed milk powder (for sauces, etc.); cheap saccharine tablets (for cooking); soy sauce (for rice and salads); lemon juice; Worcestershire sauce; Marmite, Bovril and Oxo cubes; tinned tomatoes; baked beans; cornflour (for thickening); and a variety of herbs and spices. A non-stick saucepan, frying pan and wok are invaluable.

'Will I definitely lose weight and inches if I follow these guidelines?'

Well, you should. But if you're not progressing fast enough for your liking, do refer back to my *Complete Hip and Thigh Diet* for menu guidance.

NOTE TO MANUFACTURERS

Rosemary Conley's Guide to Fat in Food is under constant revision. If your products do not appear in these tables at present, and you would like them to be included, please write to:

Nancy Webber
Rosemary Conley's Guide to Fat in Food
Grafton Books
8 Grafton Street
London
W1X 3LA.

Acknowledgements

I would like to convey my very grateful thanks to all those who helped prepare this *Guide to Fat in Food*. My particular thanks must go to my husband, Mike, who wrote to so many manufacturers asking for the appropriate information. I would also like to thank the companies for their co-operation in not only supplying the appropriate data, but also checking the fat tables at proof stage.

I would also like to acknowledge the hard work of our secretary, Diane Stevens, and Angie Spurr in the later stages. But particular thanks must go to Angela Johnson of J.V.F. Consultants Ltd. who so painstakingly collated all the data. This was an enormous task and Angela's interest and enthusiasm helped us all see the job completed.

Grams per 25g/1oz (approx)	1	2	3	4	5	6	7	8	9	10	11	12	13	14	15	16	17	18	19	20	21	22	23	24	25

ALCOHOL – GENERAL

Beers

	1	2	3	4	5	6	7	8	9	10	11	12	13	14	15	16	17	18	19	20	21	22	23	24	25
Brown Ale	♦																								
Canned Beer	♦																								
Draught	♦																								
Keg	♦																								
Lager	♦																								
Pale Ale	♦																								
Stout	♦																								
Stout, Extra	♦																								
Strong Ale	♦																								

Ciders

	1	2	3	4	5	6	7	8	9	10	11	12	13	14	15	16	17	18	19	20	21	22	23	24	25
All types	♦																								

Liqueurs

	1	2	3	4	5	6	7	8	9	10	11	12	13	14	15	16	17	18	19	20	21	22	23	24	25
Advocaat	■	■																							
Cherry Brandy	♦																								

Curacao	◆																
Spirits All types	◆																
Vermouths All types	◆																
Wines All types	◆																
Wines, Fortified Port Sherry	◆ ◆																
BAKING PRODUCTS - GENERAL Baking Powder Gelatine Yeast, Baker's Yeast, Dried	◆ ◆ ◆ ■																

2

◆ = negligible

Grams per 25g/1oz (approx)	1	2	3	4	5	6	7	8	9	10	11	12	13	14	15	16	17	18	19	20	21	22	23	24	25

RHM GROCERY (ROBERTSONS)

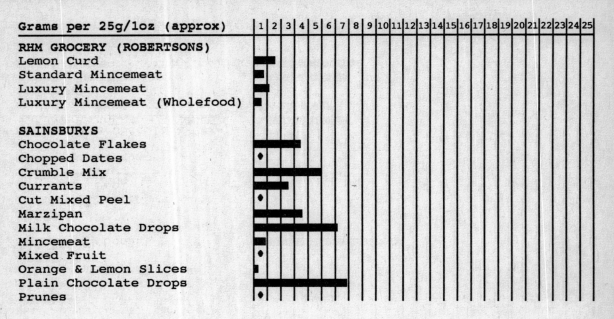

Lemon Curd	▮ (≈2)
Standard Mincemeat	▮ (≈1)
Luxury Mincemeat	▮ (≈1.5)
Luxury Mincemeat (Wholefood)	▮ (≈0.5)

SAINSBURYS

Chocolate Flakes	≈4
Chopped Dates	◆ (≈0.5)
Crumble Mix	≈5
Currants	≈3
Cut Mixed Peel	◆ (≈0.5)
Marzipan	≈4
Milk Chocolate Drops	≈7
Mincemeat	≈1
Mixed Fruit	◆ (≈0.5)
Orange & Lemon Slices	≈0.5
Plain Chocolate Drops	≈7.5
Prunes	◆ (≈0.5)

3

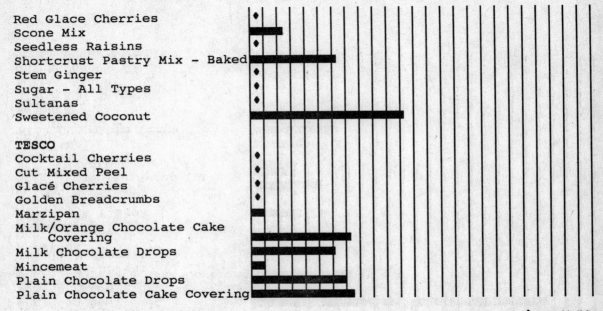

Red Glace Cherries	♦
Scone Mix	
Seedless Raisins	♦
Shortcrust Pastry Mix – Baked	
Stem Ginger	♦
Sugar – All Types	♦
Sultanas	♦
Sweetened Coconut	

TESCO

Cocktail Cherries	♦
Cut Mixed Peel	♦
Glacé Cherries	♦
Golden Breadcrumbs	♦
Marzipan	
Milk/Orange Chocolate Cake Covering	
Milk Chocolate Drops	
Mincemeat	
Plain Chocolate Drops	
Plain Chocolate Cake Covering	

♦ = negligible

Grams per 25g/1oz (approx)	1	2	3	4	5	6	7	8	9	10	11	12	13	14	15	16	17	18	19	20	21	22	23	24	25
Shredded Beef Suet																						22			
Tomato Puree	▪																								
White Chocolate Cake Covering							8																		
WAITROSE																									
Cut Mixed Peel	♦																								
Glace Cherries	♦																								
Glace Fruits	♦																								
Golden Marzipan				4																					
Stem Ginger in Syrup	♦																								
White Marzipan				4																					
BEANS, LENTILS & PULSES –																									
GENERAL																									
Baked Beans	♦																								
Black Eye Beans	♦																								
Butter Beans	♦																								
Chick Peas	▪																								
Continental Lentils	♦																								

Green Split Peas	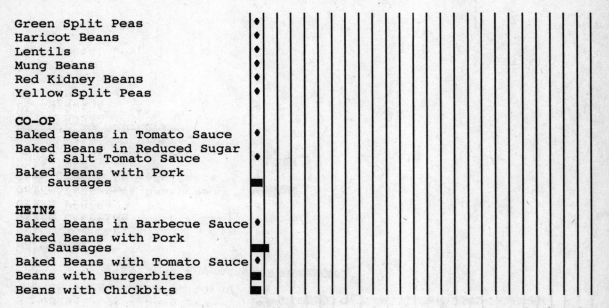
Haricot Beans	
Lentils	
Mung Beans	
Red Kidney Beans	
Yellow Split Peas	
CO-OP	
Baked Beans in Tomato Sauce	
Baked Beans in Reduced Sugar & Salt Tomato Sauce	
Baked Beans with Pork Sausages	
HEINZ	
Baked Beans in Barbecue Sauce	
Baked Beans with Pork Sausages	
Baked Beans with Tomato Sauce	
Beans with Burgerbites	
Beans with Chickbits	

♦ = negligible

Grams per 25g/1oz (approx)	1	2	3	4	5	6	7	8	9	10	11	12	13	14	15	16	17	18	19	20	21	22	23	24	25
Beans with Mini Sausages	██																								
Curried Beans with Sultanas	▍																								

MARKS & SPENCER

	1	2	3	4	5	6	7	8	9	10	11	12	13	14	15	16	17	18	19	20	21	22	23	24	25
Baked Beans - Tomato	▍																								

NESTLE (CROSSE & BLACKWELL)

	1	2	3	4	5	6	7	8	9	10	11	12	13	14	15	16	17	18	19	20	21	22	23	24	25
Baked Beans	◆																								
Beans with Beef Sausages	██																								
Fred Bear Beans and Pasta Shapes	◆																								
Beans with Pork Sausages	██																								
Beans with Hamburgers	█▌																								
Beans - No Saccharin	◆																								
Beans with Low Fat Pork Sausage	█▌																								

TESCO

Bean Salad	♦
Beans in Tomato Sauce	♦
Beans (50% Less Added Sugar and Salt)	♦
Beans with 4 Pork Sausages	▮
Beans with 8 Pork Sausages	▮
Black Eye Beans	♦
Butter Beans	♦
Chick Peas	▮
Chilli Beans	♦
Continental Lentils	♦
Green Split Peas	♦
Haricot Beans	♦
Lentils	♦
Mung Beans	♦
Red Kidney Beans	♦
Yellow Split Peas	♦

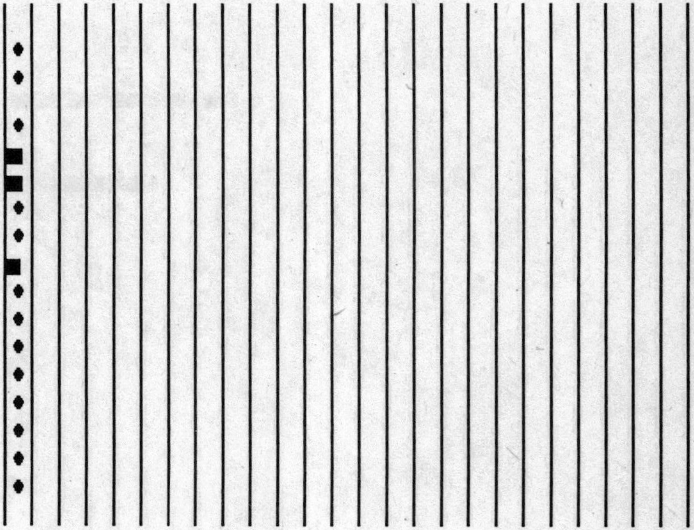

♦ = negligible

8

Grams per 25g/1oz (approx)	1	2	3	4	5	6	7	8	9	10	11	12	13	14	15	16	17	18	19	20	21	22	23	24	25

WAITROSE

Blackeye Beans – when cooked	∎																								
Broth Mix – when cooked	♦																								
Butter Beans	♦																								
Chick Peas – when cooked	∎																								
Haricot Beans	♦																								
Large Green Lentils	♦																								
Marrowfat Peas – when cooked	♦																								
Red Kidney Beans – when cooked	♦																								
Split Yellow Peas	♦																								

BEVERAGES HOT & COLD – GENERAL

Bournvita	▬																								
Cocoa Powder	▬	▬	▬	▬	▬	▬																			
Coffee	♦																								
Coffee and Chicory Essence	♦																								
Coffee Whitener	▬	▬	▬	▬	▬	▬	▬	▬	▬																

Drinking Chocolate
Horlicks
Ovaltine
Tea

BOOTS
Chocolate Malted Drink
Decaffeinated Coffee
Fat Reduced Drinking
    Chocolate
Instant Chocolate Malted
    Drink
Instant Malted Drink
Instant Hot Chocolate Drink
Malted Drink

MARKS & SPENCER
Aroma Rich Instant Coffee
Dark Roast Filter Coffee
Decaffeinated Instant Coffee

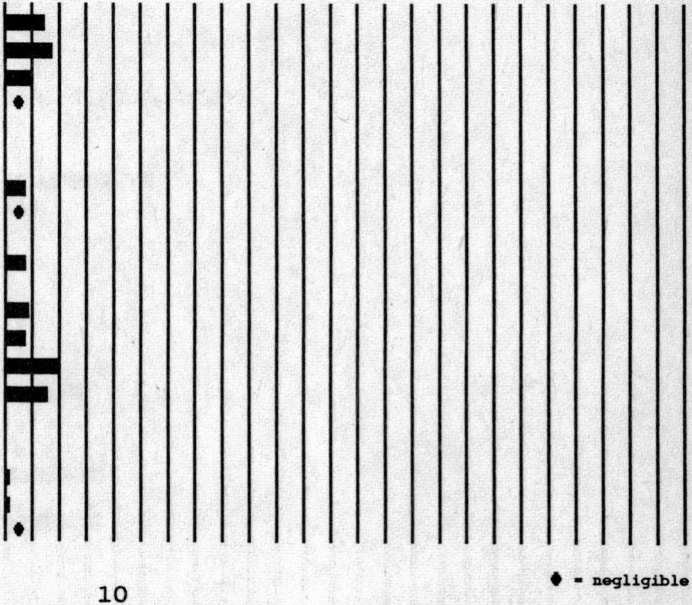

◆ = negligible

Grams per 25g/1oz (approx)	1	2	3	4	5	6	7	8	9	10	11	12	13	14	15	16	17	18	19	20	21	22	23	24	25
Fine Flavour Freeze Dried Coffee	◆																								
Fresh Ground Dark Roast Coffee	██	██	██	██																					
Fresh Ground Medium Roast Coffee	██	██	██	██																					
Instant Coffee Granules	◆																								
New Instant Coffee Granules	▌																								
One Cup Coffee Filters	██	██	██																						
Ceylon Loose Tea	▌																								
Ceylon Tea Bags	▌																								
Fine Flavour Tea Bags	▌																								
Strong Flavour Tea Bags	▌																								
Kenya Loose Tea	▌																								
Kenya Tea Bags	▌																								
One Cup Tea Bags	▌																								

11

NESTLE

Nestlé Nesquik - Strawberry

Nestlé Nesquik - Banana

Nestlé Nesquik - Chocolate

Nesquik Thick Shake -
    Chocolate

Carnation Chocolate Drink -
    Low Fat

Carnation Chocolate Drink -
    No Added Sugar

Slender Slim Choc Luxury

Slender Slim Choc Mocha

Milk Chocolate Flavoured
    Malt Drink

Nescafé High Roast

Nescafé Gold Blend

Nescafé Gold Blend -
    Decaffeinated

Santa Rica

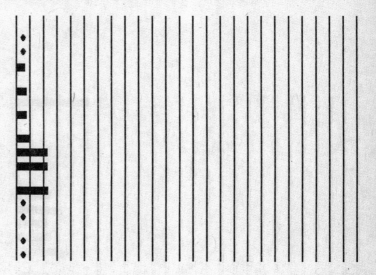

◆ = negligible

12

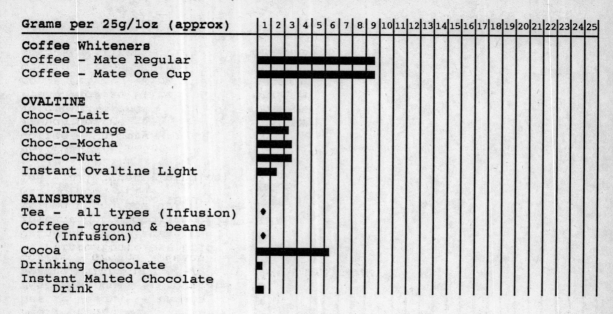

Grams per 25g/1oz (approx)	1	2	3	4	5	6	7	8	9	10	11	12	13	14	15	16	17	18	19	20	21	22	23	24	25
Coffee Whiteners																									
Coffee - Mate Regular																									
Coffee - Mate One Cup																									
OVALTINE																									
Choc-o-Lait																									
Choc-n-Orange																									
Choc-o-Mocha																									
Choc-o-Nut																									
Instant Ovaltine Light																									
SAINSBURYS																									
Tea - all types (Infusion)																									
Coffee - ground & beans (Infusion)																									
Cocoa																									
Drinking Chocolate																									
Instant Malted Chocolate Drink																									

13

Malted Chocolate Drink
Beefy Drink

TESCO
Coffee Whitener
Coffee - Ground & Beans
        (Infusion)
Drinking Chocolate
Instant Hot Chocolate Drink
Malted Chocolate Drink
Malted Food Drink
Tea - all types (Infusion)

WAITROSE
Coffee - Chicory
French Coffee
Colombian Blend
French Coffee Filter
Kenya Filter - Fine
Contin Filter - Fine
Mountain Filter - Fine

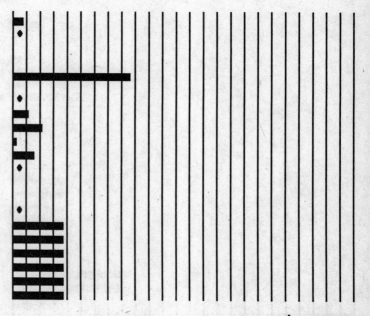

♦ = negligible

Grams per 25g/1oz (approx)	1	2	3	4	5	6	7	8	9	10	11	12	13	14	15	16	17	18	19	20	21	22	23	24	25
Kenya Ground	■	■	■	■																					
Continental Ground	■	■	■	■																					
Viennese Coffee Ground	■	■	■	■																					
Kenya Beans	■	■	■	■																					
Continental Beans	■	■	■	■																					
Colombian Beans	■	■	■	■																					
French Coffee Beans	■	■	■	■																					
Connoisseurs Coffee	■	■	■	■																					
Colombian Coffee Bags	■	■	■	■																					
Decaffeinated Coffee	■	■	■	■																					
Mild Powder	◆																								
Full Flavour Powder	◆																								
Med Granules	◆																								
Dark Granules	◆																								
Rich Roast Granules	◆																								
Mountain Freeze-Dried Coffee	◆																								
Contin Freeze-Dried Coffee	◆																								
Supreme Freeze-Dried Coffee	◆																								
Decaf Freeze-Dried Coffee	◆																								

Tea Caddy
Strong Blend Tea
Strong Blend Tea Bags
Taste of Kenya
Taste of Assam
Assam Tea
Ceylon Tea
Earl Grey Tea
Darjeeling Tea
Lapsang Tea

BISCUITS, SWEET - GENERAL
Chocolate, full coated
Cream Biscuits
Digestive, Plain
Digestive, Chocolate
Garibaldi
Ginger Nuts
Jaffa Cakes
Matzo
Muesli Biscuits

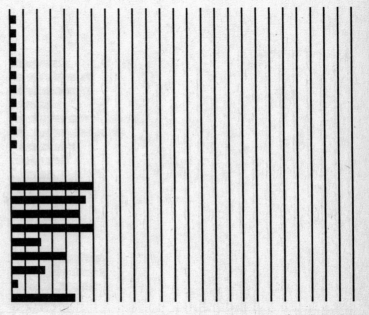

♦ - negligible

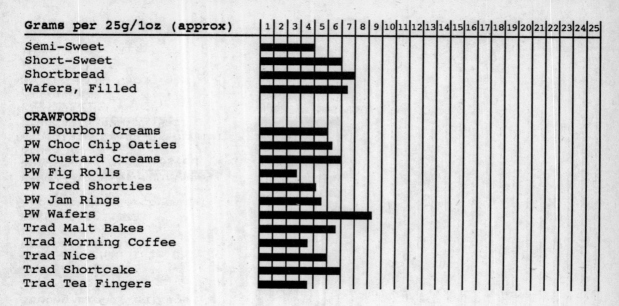

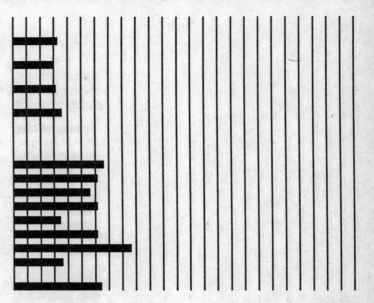

LYONS & TETLEY
Apple & Hazelnut Cereal Bar
Apricot & Chocolate Chip
    Cereal Bar
Milk Choc Chip & Raisin
    Cereal Bar
Orange & Chocolate Chip
    Cereal Bar

MARKS & SPENCER
All Butter Shortbread
    Assortment
Fancy Biscuit Assortment
Speciality Assortment
Break In
Chocolate Cream Assortment
Crunchy Sandwich Bars
Florentines
Jaffa Cakes
Malted Milk Chocolate
    Sandwich Bar

♦ = negligible

18

Grams per 25g/1oz (approx)	1 2 3 4 5 6 7 8 9 10 11 12 13 14 15 16 17 18 19 20 21 22 23 24 25
Milk Chocolate Fruit & Nut Cereal Bars	███████
Milk Chocolate Currant Topped Caramel Wafer	██████
Milk Chocolate Digestive Biscuits	██████
Milk Chocolate Orange Biscuit	███████
Milk Chocolate Caramel Wafer	██████
Milk Chocolate Crunch	██████
Milk Chocolate Oat Crunchies	██████
Milk Chocolate Sandwich	██████
Milk Chocolate Tea Cakes	████
Plain Chocolate Digestive	███████
Plain Chocolate Ginger Biscuits	██████
Plain Chocolate Mint Sandwich Bars	███████
Plain Chocolate Biscuit Thins	█████
Plain Chocolate Crunchies	██████

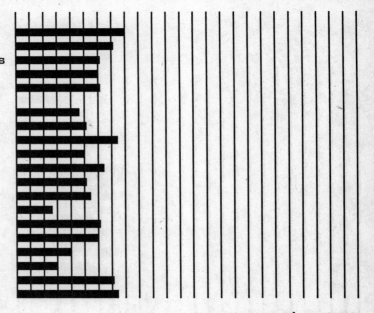

Swiss Milk Chocolate Hazelnut Biscuits	
Take 4	
Choc Chip & Hazelnut Cookies	
Chocolate Chip Cookies	
Trad Choc Chip Cookies	
Trad All Butter Sultana Cookies	
Trad Oatflake Cookies	
Viennese Chocolate Sandwich	
Bourbon Creams	
Butter Crunch Creams	
Fruit and Nut Creams	
Rich Tea Finger Creams	
Bran Sunnywheat Crackers	
Butter Puff	
Butterfly Crackers	
Apple Crumble Cookies	
Black Cherry Tartlets	
Break	
Luxury Petit Four Biscuits	

♦ = negligible

Grams per 25g/1oz (approx)	1	2	3	4	5	6	7	8	9	10	11	12	13	14	15	16	17	18	19	20	21	22	23	24	25

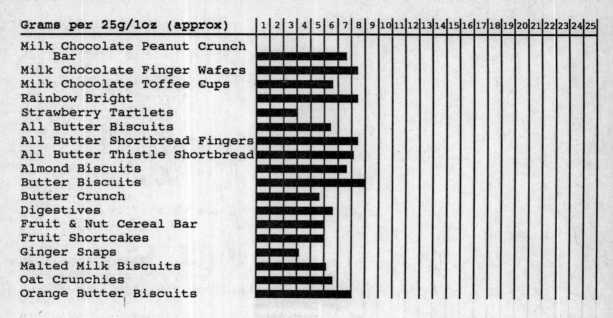

Milk Chocolate Peanut Crunch Bar
Milk Chocolate Finger Wafers
Milk Chocolate Toffee Cups
Rainbow Bright
Strawberry Tartlets
All Butter Biscuits
All Butter Shortbread Fingers
All Butter Thistle Shortbread
Almond Biscuits
Butter Biscuits
Butter Crunch
Digestives
Fruit & Nut Cereal Bar
Fruit Shortcakes
Ginger Snaps
Malted Milk Biscuits
Oat Crunchies
Orange Butter Biscuits

Rich Tea
Rich Tea Finger
Round Shorties
Shortbread Petticoat Tails
Shortcake
Wheaten Sweetmeal

McVITIES
5 4 3 2 1
Abbey Crunch
Arrowroot
Butter Puffs (Crawfords)
Choc Chip & Hazelnut Cookies
Choc Chip & Orange Cookies
Chocolate Homewheat
Balmoral Shortbread
Highland Fingers
Petticoat Tails
Traditional Malties
Digestive
Digestive Creams

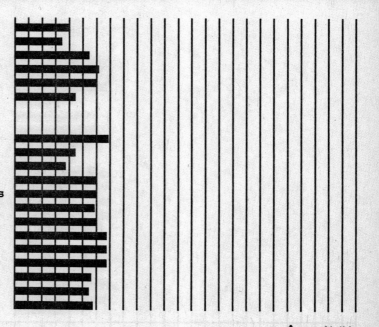

◆ = negligible

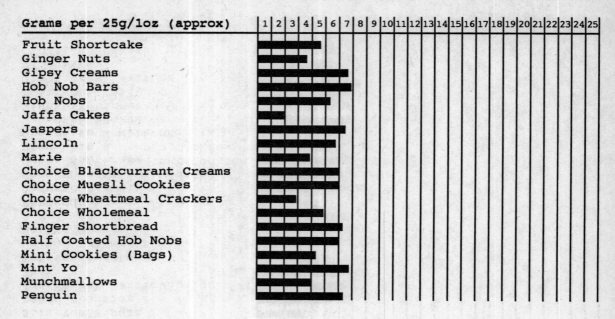

Grams per 25g/1oz (approx)	1	2	3	4	5	6	7	8	9	10	11	12	13	14	15	16	17	18	19	20	21	22	23	24	25
Fruit Shortcake																									
Ginger Nuts																									
Gipsy Creams																									
Hob Nob Bars																									
Hob Nobs																									
Jaffa Cakes																									
Jaspers																									
Lincoln																									
Marie																									
Choice Blackcurrant Creams																									
Choice Muesli Cookies																									
Choice Wheatmeal Crackers																									
Choice Wholemeal																									
Finger Shortbread																									
Half Coated Hob Nobs																									
Mini Cookies (Bags)																									
Mint Yo																									
Munchmallows																									
Penguin																									

Rich Tea
Solar Choc Chip
Solar Tropical Fruit
Sports
Taxi
Toffee Yo
United Golden Crunch
United Orange

NABISCO
Coconut Biscuit
Choc Chip N' Nut Cookie
Dutch Shortcake
Digestive
Digestive – Milk Chocolate
    Half Coated
Digestive – Plain Chocolate
    Half Coated
Lemon Puff
Romany
Sponge Finger

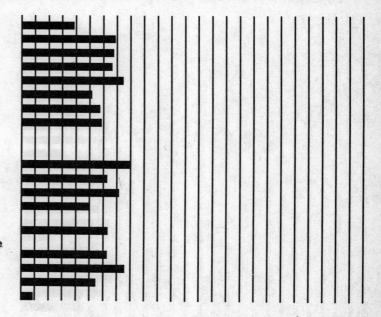

♦ = negligible

Grams per 25g/1oz (approx)	1	2	3	4	5	6	7	8	9	10	11	12	13	14	15	16	17	18	19	20	21	22	23	24	25
Bath Oliver																									
Chocolate Oliver																									
Folies																									
Folies Au Chocolate																									
Bourbon																									
Coconut Mallows																									
Coffee Creams																									
Custard Creams																									
Coated Mallows - Milk																									
Coated Mallows - Orange																									
Iced Gem																									
Jamboree Mallows																									
Lincoln																									
Megabar																									
Nice Creams																									
Nice																									
Neapolitan Wafers																									
Rich Tea																									
Rich Osborne																									

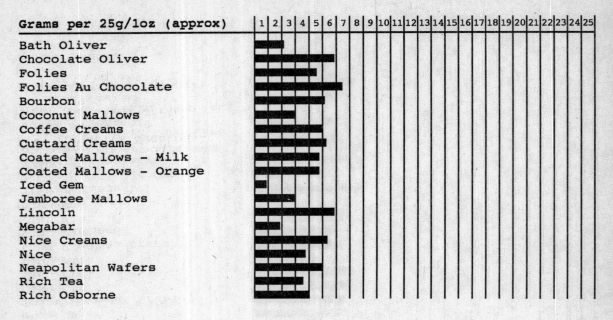

Shortcake
Snow Balls
Snack Cookies – Choc Chip
Club Coffee
Club Fruit
Club Milk
Club Orange
Club Plain
Club Mint
Fig Roll
Trio

TESCO
Economy Milk Chocolate
    Digestive Sweetmeal
Jaffa Cakes
Milk Chocolate Caramel
    Coated Wafers
Milk Chocolate Caramel
    Shortcake

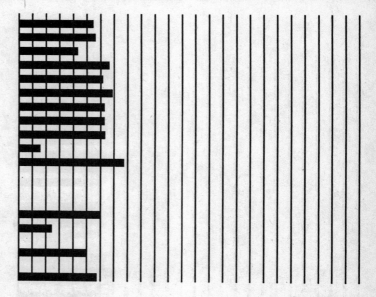

26

◆ = negligible

Grams per 25g/1oz (approx)	value (approx, squares)
Milk Chocolate Coated Mint Wafer Fingers	7
Milk Chocolate Coated Wafer Fingers	7½
Milk Chocolate Digestive	7
Milk Chocolate Digestive Sweetmeal	7
Milk Chocolate Fruit and Nut	7
Milk Chocolate Muesli	7
Milk Chocolate Orange Sandwich	7
Milk Chocolate Sandwich	7
Milk Chocolate Shortcake	7
Milk Chocolate Teacakes	5–7
Milk Chocolate Wafers	7
Plain Chocolate Digestive Sweetmeal	7
Caramel Cookie Rings	6
Choc Chip Shortbread	7

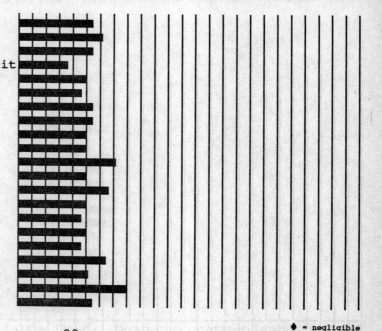

Chocolate Chip
Economy Chocolate Chip
Honey and Oatmeal
Mini Chocolate Chip and Fruit
Mini Chocolate Chip and Nut
Muesli
Stem Ginger
Sultana
Bakewell Creams
Bourbon Creams
Coconut Crumble Creams
Coffee Creams
Currant Crunch Creams
Custard Creams
Economy Bourbon Creams
Economy Custard Creams
Ginger Crunch Creams
Golden Crunch Creams
Jam and Cream Sandwich
Lemon Puffs
Malted Milk Creams

♦ = negligible

Grams per 25g/1oz (approx)

Biscuit	Grams per 25g/1oz (approx)
Orange Creams	5
Strawberry Crumble Creams	6.5
Treacle Crunch Creams	6.5
All Butter Fruit	6
All Butter Shortcake	6
All Butter Thins	5
Almond Shorties	7
Coconut Macaroons	7.5
Coconut Rings	7.5
Digestive	6.5
Economy Digestive	7
Economy Fruit Shortcake	6.5
Economy Rich Tea	5
Economy Shortcake	6
Fruit Shortcake	6.5
Garibaldi	2.5
Ginger Nuts	2.5
Lemon Crisp	5
Lincoln	6.5

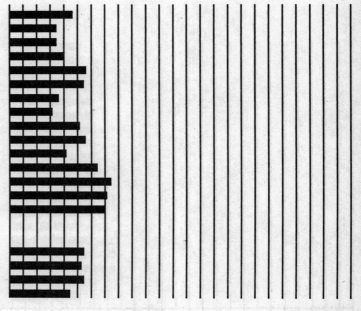

Malted Milk
Marie
Morning Coffee
Nice
Peanut Crunch
Rich Shortie
Rich Tea
Rich Tea Fingers
Shortcake
Snowballs
Spicy Fruit Crunch
Petticoat Tails
Shortbread Fingers
Thistle Shortbread
Wholemeal Shortbread Fingers

WAITROSE
Highland Shorties
Coconut Rings
Muesli Cookies
Petit Beurre

♦ = negligible

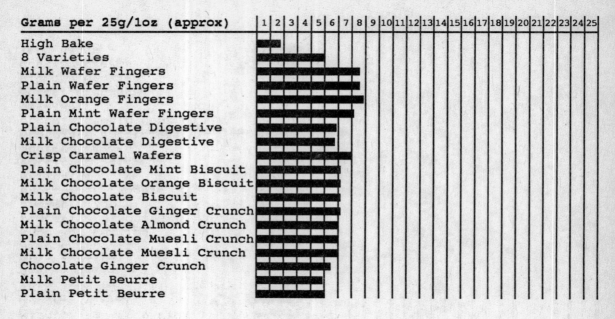

Grams per 25g/1oz (approx)	1	2	3	4	5	6	7	8	9	10	11	12	13	14	15	16	17	18	19	20	21	22	23	24	25
High Bake																									
8 Varieties																									
Milk Wafer Fingers																									
Plain Wafer Fingers																									
Milk Orange Fingers																									
Plain Mint Wafer Fingers																									
Plain Chocolate Digestive																									
Milk Chocolate Digestive																									
Crisp Caramel Wafers																									
Plain Chocolate Mint Biscuit																									
Milk Chocolate Orange Biscuit																									
Milk Chocolate Biscuit																									
Plain Chocolate Ginger Crunch																									
Milk Chocolate Almond Crunch																									
Plain Chocolate Muesli Crunch																									
Milk Chocolate Muesli Crunch																									
Chocolate Ginger Crunch																									
Milk Petit Beurre																									
Plain Petit Beurre																									

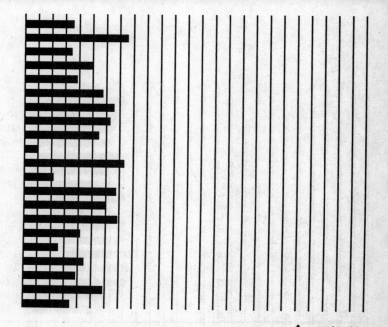

Rich Tea Biscuits
Wafer Sandwich 6 Pack
Tea Fingers
Fruit Shortcake
Nice Biscuits
Butter Biscuits
Almond Biscuits
Choc-Nut Cookies
Digestive Biscuits
Sponge Fingers
Shortbread Fingers
Garibaldi
Petticoat Tails
Shortcake
Chocolate Shortbread
Chocolate Chip Cookies
Cafe Noir
Butter Crunch
Crunchy Cookies
Custard Creams
Iced Rings

♦ = negligible

Grams per 25g/1oz (approx)

Biscuit	Grams per 25g/1oz (approx)
Bourbon	6
Jam Creams	6
Ginger Snaps	3
Ginger Thins	4½
Chocolate & Orange Cookies	6
Coconut Cookies	6
Malted Milk Biscuits	6
Ginger Cookies	6
Hazelnut Cookies	7
Oatflake & Honey Cookies	6
Treacle Cookies	7
Sultana & Spice Cookies	6½
Crunchy Creams	6
Treacle Creams	6½
Ginger Creams	6
Coconut Crumble Creams	7
Digestive Finger Creams	6

BISCUITS, SAVOURY - GENERAL

Cream Crackers

Crispbread, Rye

Crispbread, Wheat Starch
    Reduced

Oatcakes

Water Biscuits

Wheat Crackers

MARKS & SPENCER

Bran Sunnywheat Crackers

Butter Puff

Butterfly Crackers

Cheese Bites

Cheese Sandwich

Cheese Snaps

Cheese Straws

Cheese Thins

Herb Thins

Onion Kites

High Bake Water Biscuits

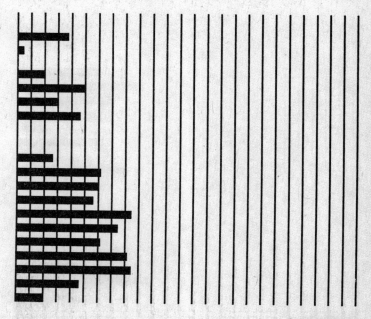

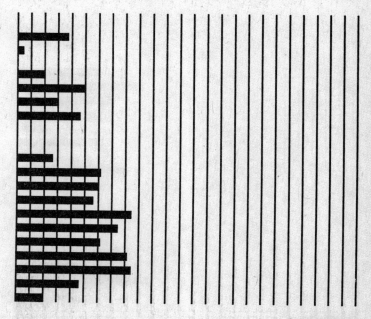

♦ = negligible

Grams per 25g/1oz (approx)	1	2	3	4	5	6	7	8	9	10	11	12	13	14	15	16	17	18	19	20	21	22	23	24	25

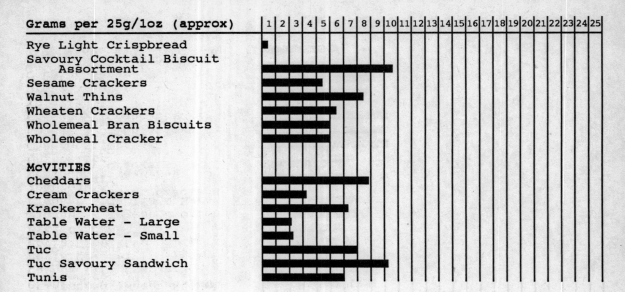

Rye Light Crispbread

Savoury Cocktail Biscuit
    Assortment

Sesame Crackers

Walnut Thins

Wheaten Crackers

Wholemeal Bran Biscuits

Wholemeal Cracker

McVITIES

Cheddars

Cream Crackers

Krackerwheat

Table Water – Large

Table Water – Small

Tuc

Tuc Savoury Sandwich

Tunis

35

NABISCO

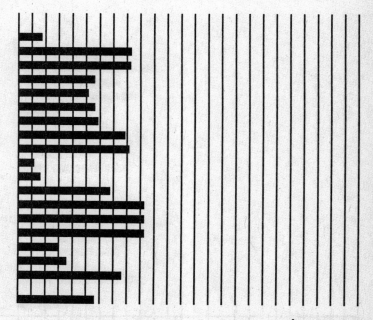

High Bake Water Biscuits
Cheese Sandwich
Cheese & Onion Sandwich
Cheese Ritz Cracker
Hovis Cracker
Hovis Digestive
Ritz Cracker
Piquant - Cheese & Onion
Piquant - Garlic & Herbs
Teabreak
Wholewheat Teabreak
Cheeselets
Cheese Sticks
Cheese & Onion Sticks
Cheese & Tomato Sticks
Twiglets
Cream Cracker
Cornish Wafer
Farmhouse - Brown Wheat
    Crackers

◆ = negligible

Grams per 25g/1oz (approx)	1	2	3	4	5	6	7	8	9	10	11	12	13	14	15	16	17	18	19	20	21	22	23	24	25

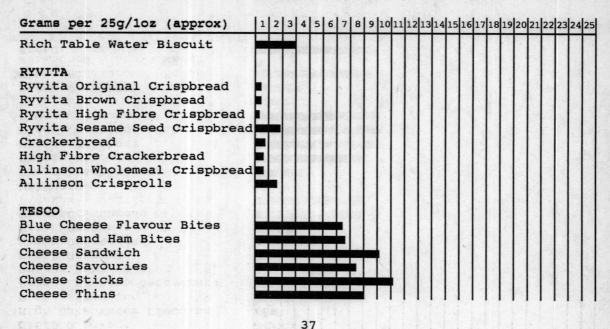

Rich Table Water Biscuit — 3

RYVITA
Ryvita Original Crispbread — 0.5
Ryvita Brown Crispbread — 0.5
Ryvita High Fibre Crispbread — 0.5
Ryvita Sesame Seed Crispbread — 2
Crackerbread — 1
High Fibre Crackerbread — 1
Allinson Wholemeal Crispbread — 0.5
Allinson Crisprolls — 2

TESCO
Blue Cheese Flavour Bites — 7
Cheese and Ham Bites — 7
Cheese Sandwich — 9
Cheese Savouries — 8
Cheese Sticks — 10
Cheese Thins — 8

Cream Crackers
High Bake Water Biscuits
Pizza Crackers
Poppy and Sesame Crackers
Rye Crispbread
Snack Crackers
Wheat Crackers
Wheat Crackers with Bran
Wheat Crispbread

WAITROSE
Cream Cracker
Cheese Sandwich
Sesame Crackers
Wheat Crackers
Savoury Crackers

<u>**BREAD - GENERAL**</u>
Wholemeal, Brown, Hovis,
    White
Fried

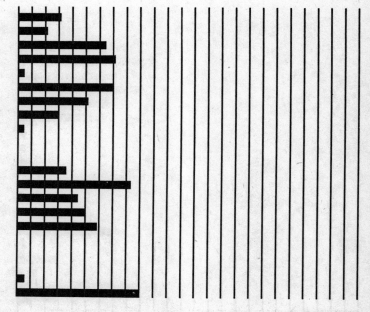

◆ = negligible

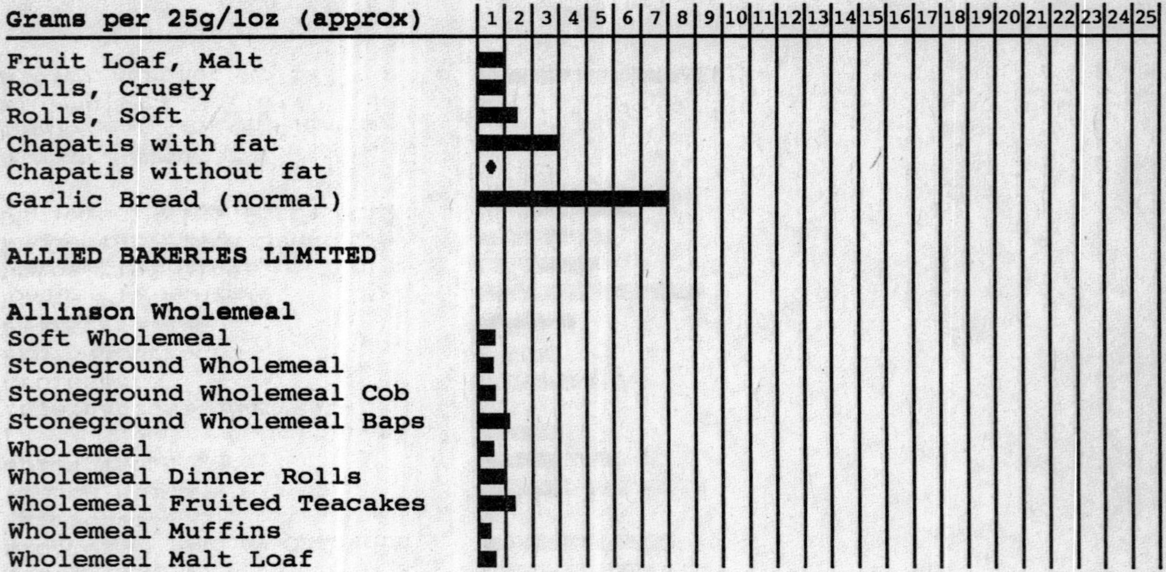

Grams per 25g/1oz (approx)	1	2	3	4	5	6	7	8	9	10	11	12	13	14	15	16	17	18	19	20	21	22	23	24	25

Fruit Loaf, Malt
Rolls, Crusty
Rolls, Soft
Chapatis with fat
Chapatis without fat
Garlic Bread (normal)

ALLIED BAKERIES LIMITED

Allinson Wholemeal
Soft Wholemeal
Stoneground Wholemeal
Stoneground Wholemeal Cob
Stoneground Wholemeal Baps
Wholemeal
Wholemeal Dinner Rolls
Wholemeal Fruited Teacakes
Wholemeal Muffins
Wholemeal Malt Loaf

39

Wholemeal Snack Roll

Crust Gold
Bloomer
Farmhouse
French Stick
Split Tin

International Harvest
Croissants
Fruited Brioche
Plain Brioche
White Pitta Bread
White Mini Pitta
Wholemeal Pitta Bread
Wholemeal Mini Pitta Bread

Mighty White
Mighty White Bread
Mighty Bite Rolls
Mighty Muncher Rolls

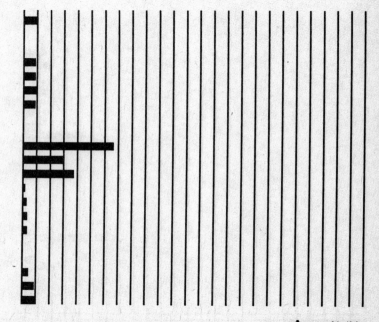

40

♦ = negligible

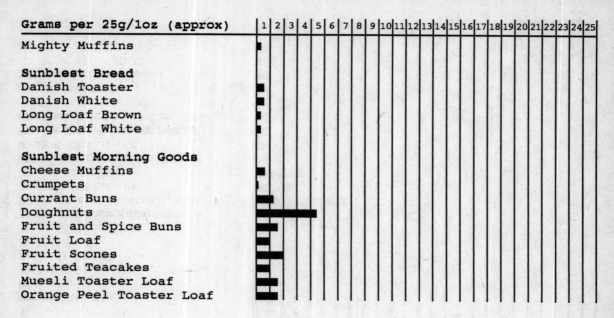

Grams per 25g/1oz (approx) — scale 1 2 3 4 5 6 7 8 9 10 11 12 13 14 15 16 17 18 19 20 21 22 23 24 25

Mighty Muffins

Sunblest Bread
Danish Toaster
Danish White
Long Loaf Brown
Long Loaf White

Sunblest Morning Goods
Cheese Muffins
Crumpets
Currant Buns
Doughnuts
Fruit and Spice Buns
Fruit Loaf
Fruit Scones
Fruited Teacakes
Muesli Toaster Loaf
Orange Peel Toaster Loaf

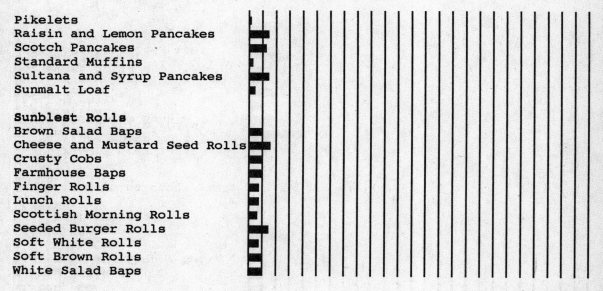

Pikelets
Raisin and Lemon Pancakes
Scotch Pancakes
Standard Muffins
Sultana and Syrup Pancakes
Sunmalt Loaf

Sunblest Rolls
Brown Salad Baps
Cheese and Mustard Seed Rolls
Crusty Cobs
Farmhouse Baps
Finger Rolls
Lunch Rolls
Scottish Morning Rolls
Seeded Burger Rolls
Soft White Rolls
Soft Brown Rolls
White Salad Baps

♦ = negligible

Grams per 25g/1oz (approx)	1	2	3	4	5	6	7	8	9	10	11	12	13	14	15	16	17	18	19	20	21	22	23	24	25

Vitbe

HiBran Bread	▓																								
HiBran Rolls	▓																								
HiBran Fruit & Honey Malt Loaf	▓																								
Raisin Bran	▓	▓	▓																						
Harvester Bread	▓																								
Wheatgerm Bread	▓																								

BOOTS

Country Rolls	▓																								
Country Loaf	▓																								
Extra Fibre White Loaf	▓																								
Extra Fibre White Rolls	▓																								
Shapers Loaf	▓																								
Shapers Rolls	▓																								
Wholemeal Bread	▓																								
Wholemeal Rolls	▓																								
Wholemeal Scones	▓	▓	▓																						

MARKS & SPENCER

Brown
Allinson Wholemeal Bread
Hi-Bran Loaf
Hovis Loaf
Mixed Grain Loaf
Multi Grain Bread
Stoneground Wholemeal Loaf
Vitbe - Wheatgerm Bread
Wholemeal Picnic Mini Pittas
Wholemeal Sandwich Bread

White
Batched White Loaf
Soft Grain White Loaf
Picnic Mini Pittas
Crusty Bread
Garlic Baguette

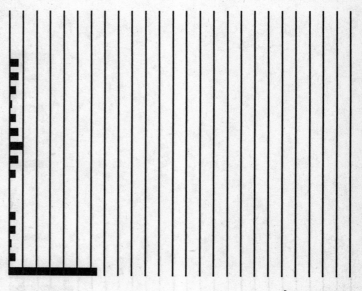

44

♦ = negligible

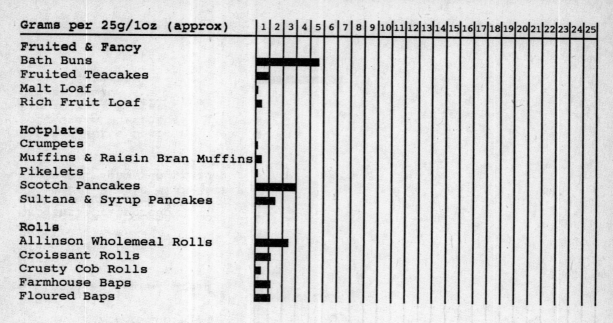

Grams per 25g/1oz (approx)	1	2	3	4	5	6	7	8	9	10	11	12	13	14	15	16	17	18	19	20	21	22	23	24	25

Fruited & Fancy
Bath Buns
Fruited Teacakes
Malt Loaf
Rich Fruit Loaf

Hotplate
Crumpets
Muffins & Raisin Bran Muffins
Pikelets
Scotch Pancakes
Sultana & Syrup Pancakes

Rolls
Allinson Wholemeal Rolls
Croissant Rolls
Crusty Cob Rolls
Farmhouse Baps
Floured Baps

Hi-Bran Baps	
Old English and Scottish Rolls	
Aberdeen Rolls	
Fruited Treacle Crumpets	
Potato Scones	
Square Loaf	
RYVITA	
Original Crispbread	
Dark Rye Crispbread	
Sesame Crispbread	
High Fibre Crispbread	
TESCO	
Bran Loaf	
Brown	
Crusty Bread - all types	
Danish Loaf	
Fruit Batch	
Fruit Loaf	

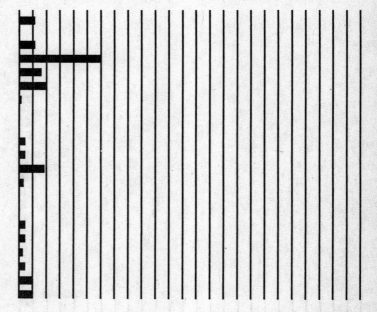

♦ = negligible

Grams per 25g/1oz (approx)	1	2	3	4	5	6	7	8	9	10	11	12	13	14	15	16	17	18	19	20	21	22	23	24	25
Hovis	█																								
Malt Loaf	█																								
Natural White	█																								
Soft White Batch	█																								
Stoneground Wholemeal	█																								
Stoneground Wholemeal Batch	▊																								
Wheatgerm	█																								
White	█																								
Wholemeal	█																								
Bran Baps	█																								
Brown Morning Rolls	█																								
Brown Snack Rolls	█																								
Cheese Muffins	█																								
Fruit Buns	█																								
Muffins	▊																								
Natural White Rolls	█																								
Plain Cookies	█																								
Scottish Crumpets	█▌																								
Scottish Muffins	█																								

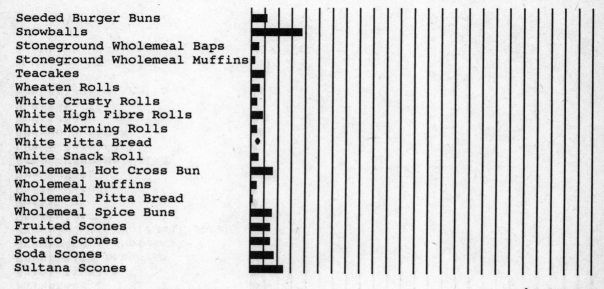

Seeded Burger Buns
Snowballs
Stoneground Wholemeal Baps
Stoneground Wholemeal Muffins
Teacakes
Wheaten Rolls
White Crusty Rolls
White High Fibre Rolls
White Morning Rolls
White Pitta Bread
White Snack Roll
Wholemeal Hot Cross Bun
Wholemeal Muffins
Wholemeal Pitta Bread
Wholemeal Spice Buns
Fruited Scones
Potato Scones
Soda Scones
Sultana Scones

48

◆ = negligible

Grams per 25g/1oz (approx)	1	2	3	4	5	6	7	8	9	10	11	12	13	14	15	16	17	18	19	20	21	22	23	24	25

BREAKFAST CEREALS – GENERAL

Food	Approx grams per 25g/1oz
All Bran	▉ (~2)
Branflakes	▉ (~1)
Cornflakes	◆ (~1)
Grapenuts	
Muesli	▉▉▉ (~3)
Oatmeal, raw	▉▉ (~2)
Porridge	▉ (~1)
Puffed Wheat	▉ (~1)
Ready Brek	▉▉▉ (~3)
Rice Krispies	▉ (~1)
Rye & Raisin	▉ (~1)
Shredded Wheat	
Special K	▉ (~1)
Sugar Puffs	◆ (~1)
Weetabix	▉ (~1)

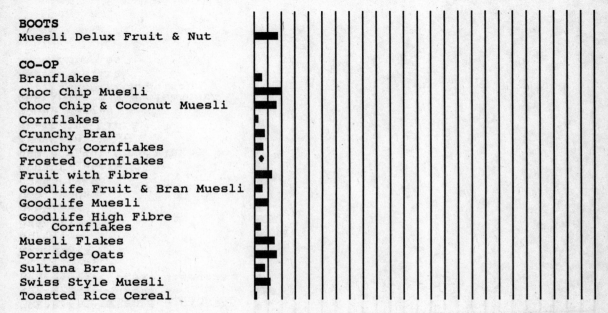

BOOTS
Muesli Delux Fruit & Nut

CO-OP
Branflakes
Choc Chip Muesli
Choc Chip & Coconut Muesli
Cornflakes
Crunchy Bran
Crunchy Cornflakes
Frosted Cornflakes
Fruit with Fibre
Goodlife Fruit & Bran Muesli
Goodlife Muesli
Goodlife High Fibre
        Cornflakes
Muesli Flakes
Porridge Oats
Sultana Bran
Swiss Style Muesli
Toasted Rice Cereal

◆ = negligible

50

Grams per 25g/1oz (approx)	1	2	3	4	5	6	7	8	9	10	11	12	13	14	15	16	17	18	19	20	21	22	23	24	25
Wheat Flakes																									
Wholewheat Muesli																									
Wholewheat Cereal Biscuits																									
KELLOGG'S																									
All-Bran																									
Bran Flakes																									
Bran Buds																									
Coco Pops																									
Corn Flakes																									
Country Store																									
Crunchy Nut Corn Flakes																									
Frosties																									
Fruit 'n' Fibre																									
Honey Smacks																									
Nutri-Grain – Wholewheat Flakes with Raisins																									
Raisin Splitz																									
Rice Krispies																									

Ricicles
Special K
Start
Sultana Bran
Summer Orchard
Toppas

MARKS & SPENCER
Bran Muesli - Unsweetened
Breakfast Special Cereal
Chocolate Flake Crunch
Tropical Fruit Crunch

**RHM GROCERY (THE SHREDDED
        WHEAT COMPANY)**
Bran Flakes
Fruit Wheats
Shredded Wheat
Shreddies
Small Shredded Wheat
Team Flakes

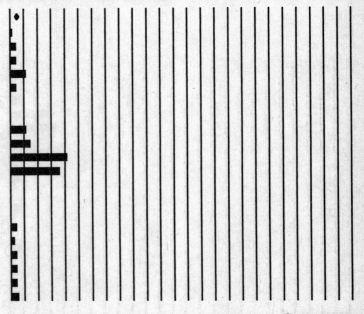

◆ = negligible

Grams per 25g/1oz (approx)	1	2	3	4	5	6	7	8	9	10	11	12	13	14	15	16	17	18	19	20	21	22	23	24	25
RYVITA																									
Cracked Wheat Flakes	▐																								
Hi-Bran Crispy Rice	▐																								
High Fibre Cornflakes	▌																								
Morning Bran	▐																								
SAINSBURYS																									
Apple Bran	▐																								
Bran Flakes	▐																								
Cocosnaps	▐																								
Cornflakes	♦																								
Crunchy Oat Cereal	███			▌																					
Crunchy Oat Cereal with Bran & Apple	███		▌																						
Deluxe Muesli	███		▌																						
Fruit & Fibre Flakes	▐																								
High Fibre Bran with Raisins	▐																								
High Fibre Bran	▐																								
Honey Nut Cornflakes	▐																								

Instant Hot Oat Cereal
Instant Hot Oat Cereal & Bran
Malted Wheats
Mini Wheats
Muesli
Natural Bran
Oat & Bran Flakes
Puffed Wheat
Rice Pops
Scotch Oat Flakes with Bran
Snowflakes
Sultana Bran
Toasted Bran
Wheat Flakes
Wholewheat Miniflakes

TESCO
Bran Flakes
Bran Flakes with Sultanas
Bran Muesli
Breakfast Bran

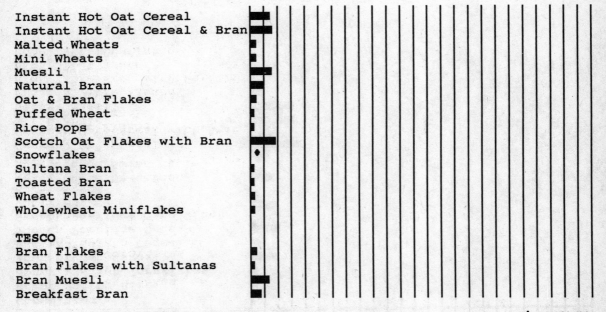

♦ = negligible

Grams per 25g/1oz (approx)	1	2	3	4	5	6	7	8	9	10	11	12	13	14	15	16	17	18	19	20	21	22	23	24	25
Cornflakes																									
Crisp Puffed Rice																									
Honey and Nut Cornflakes																									
Instant Oat Cereal																									
Rye and Raisin Cereal																									
Scotch Porridge Oats																									
Scotch Porridge Oats with Bran																									
Sugar Flakes																									
Swiss Style Breakfast																									
Unsweetened Swiss Style Muesli																									
Wholewheat Cereal																									
Wholewheat Flakes																									
Wholewheat Muesli																									

WAITROSE

	1	2	3	4	5	6	7	8	9	10	11	12	13	14	15	16	17	18	19	20	21	22	23	24	25
Bran Muesli																									
Branflakes																									

55

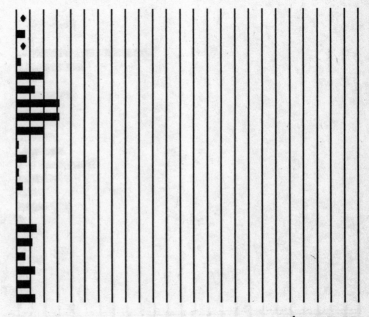

Cornflakes
Crunchy Nut Cornflakes
Frosted Cornflakes
Fruit & Fibre Muesli
Fruit & Nut Muesli
Muesli Cereal
Oat Crunchy – Almonds
Oat Crunchy – Fruits
Porridge Oats
Rice Crunchies
Wheat Bran
Wheat Flakes
Wholewheat Cereal Biscuit

WEETABIX
Alpen with Tropical Fruit
Alpen
Bran Fare
Cruesli
Honey and Fruit F.H.B.
No Added Sugar Alpen

◆ = negligible

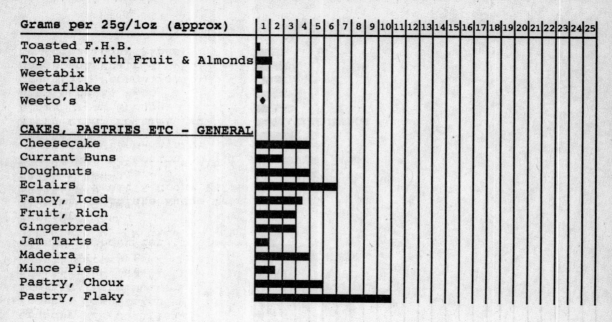

Grams per 25g/1oz (approx)	1	2	3	4	5	6	7	8	9	10	11	12	13	14	15	16	17	18	19	20	21	22	23	24	25
Toasted F.H.B.																									
Top Bran with Fruit & Almonds																									
Weetabix																									
Weetaflake																									
Weeto's																									

CAKES, PASTRIES ETC - GENERAL

	1	2	3	4	5	6	7	8	9	10	11	12	13	14	15	16	17	18	19	20	21	22	23	24	25
Cheesecake																									
Currant Buns																									
Doughnuts																									
Eclairs																									
Fancy, Iced																									
Fruit, Rich																									
Gingerbread																									
Jam Tarts																									
Madeira																									
Mince Pies																									
Pastry, Choux																									
Pastry, Flaky																									

Pastry, Shortcrust
Plain
Rock
Scones
Scotch Pancakes
Sponge with fat
Sponge without fat

ICELAND
Alabama Chocolate Fudge Cake
Assorted Fruit & Cream Puffs
Black Forest Gateau
Cheesecake Selection
Chocolate Grand-Marnier
    Gateau
Dairy Cream Eclairs
Dairy Cream Sponge
Exotic Fruit Flan
Ice Cream Sponge Rolls
Jam Doughnuts
Lemon Meringue Pie

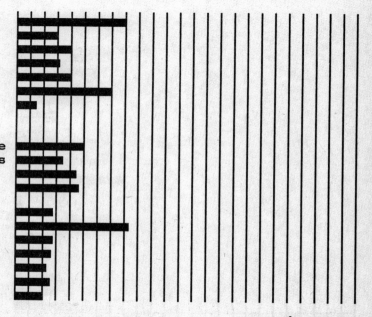

♦ = negligible

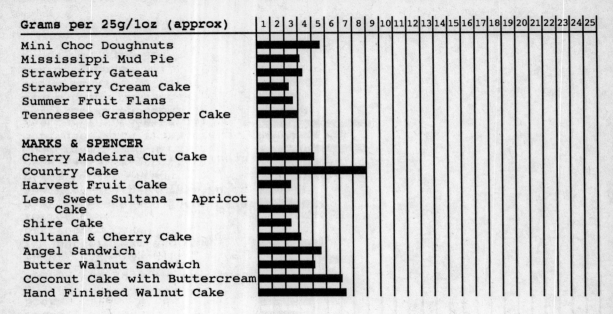

Grams per 25g/1oz (approx)	1	2	3	4	5	6	7	8	9	10	11	12	13	14	15	16	17	18	19	20	21	22	23	24	25
Mini Choc Doughnuts					■																				
Mississippi Mud Pie			■																						
Strawberry Gateau			■																						
Strawberry Cream Cake		■																							
Summer Fruit Flans			■																						
Tennessee Grasshopper Cake																									

MARKS & SPENCER

	1	2	3	4	5	6	7	8	9	10	11	12	13	14	15	16	17	18	19	20	21	22	23	24	25
Cherry Madeira Cut Cake				■																					
Country Cake								■																	
Harvest Fruit Cake		■																							
Less Sweet Sultana – Apricot Cake																									
Shire Cake			■																						
Sultana & Cherry Cake			■																						
Angel Sandwich					■																				
Butter Walnut Sandwich				■																					
Coconut Cake with Buttercream						■																			
Hand Finished Walnut Cake							■																		

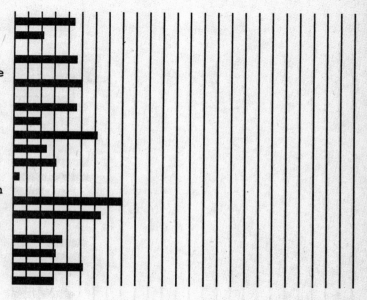

Lemon Iced Madeira Sandwich
Mothers Day Cake
Sponge Gateau with
Buttercream and Jam
Sponge Gateau with Chocolate
Buttercream
Sponge Sandwich with
Buttercream and Jam
Battenburg Cake
Toffee Cake
Parkin Cut Cake
Apple Sponge Sandwich
Fresh Cream Scones
Chocolate Eclairs with Fresh
Cream
Meringues with Fresh Cream
Raspberry Sponge Sandwich
with Fresh Cream
Baked Lemon Cheesecake
Choux Buns
Apricot Sponge Roll

60

♦ = negligible

Grams per 25g/1oz (approx)   1 2 3 4 5 6 7 8 9 10 11 12 13 14 15 16 17 18 19 20 21 22 23 24 25

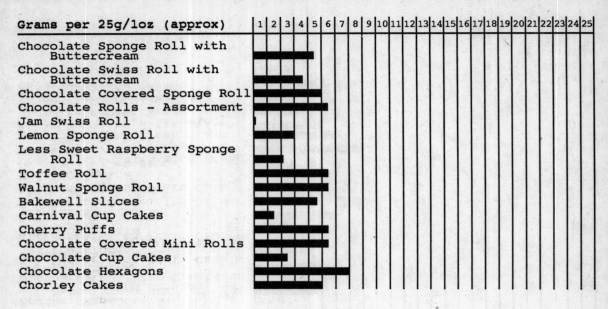

Chocolate Sponge Roll with Buttercream
Chocolate Swiss Roll with Buttercream
Chocolate Covered Sponge Roll
Chocolate Rolls - Assortment
Jam Swiss Roll
Lemon Sponge Roll
Less Sweet Raspberry Sponge Roll
Toffee Roll
Walnut Sponge Roll
Bakewell Slices
Carnival Cup Cakes
Cherry Puffs
Chocolate Covered Mini Rolls
Chocolate Cup Cakes
Chocolate Hexagons
Chorley Cakes

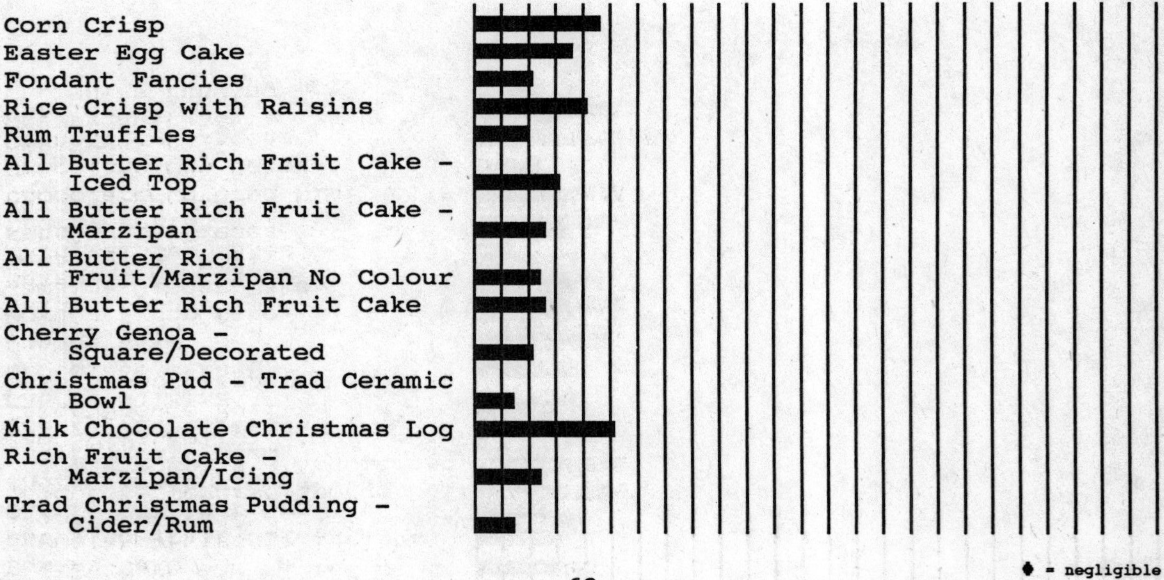

Corn Crisp

Easter Egg Cake

Fondant Fancies

Rice Crisp with Raisins

Rum Truffles

All Butter Rich Fruit Cake –
    Iced Top

All Butter Rich Fruit Cake –
    Marzipan

All Butter Rich
    Fruit/Marzipan No Colour

All Butter Rich Fruit Cake

Cherry Genoa –
    Square/Decorated

Christmas Pud – Trad Ceramic
    Bowl

Milk Chocolate Christmas Log

Rich Fruit Cake –
    Marzipan/Icing

Trad Christmas Pudding –
    Cider/Rum

♦ = negligible

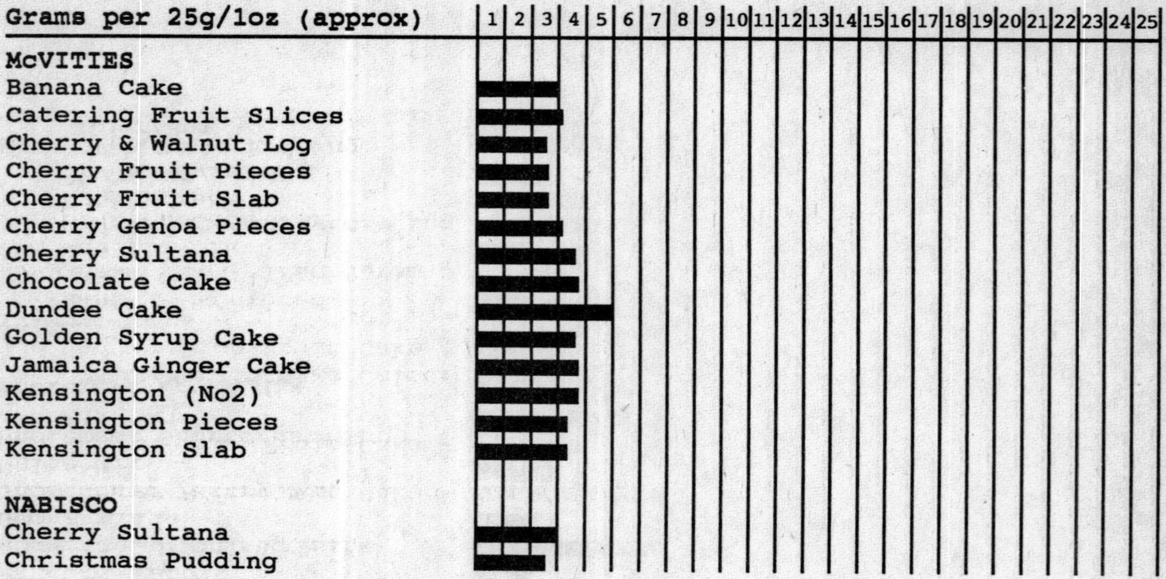

Grams per 25g/1oz (approx)	1	2	3	4	5	6	7	8	9	10	11	12	13	14	15	16	17	18	19	20	21	22	23	24	25

McVITIES
Banana Cake
Catering Fruit Slices
Cherry & Walnut Log
Cherry Fruit Pieces
Cherry Fruit Slab
Cherry Genoa Pieces
Cherry Sultana
Chocolate Cake
Dundee Cake
Golden Syrup Cake
Jamaica Ginger Cake
Kensington (No2)
Kensington Pieces
Kensington Slab

NABISCO
Cherry Sultana
Christmas Pudding

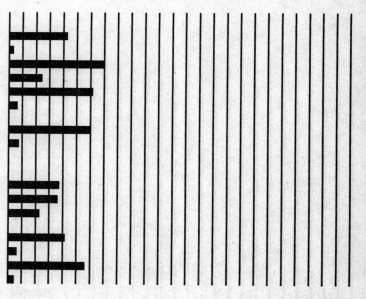

RHM GROCERY (McDOUGALLS)
Crumble Mix
Pancake Mix
Pudding & Dumpling Mix
Scone Mix
Shortcrust Pastry Mix
White Mix
Wholemeal Shortcrust Pastry
    Mix
Wholemeal Bread Mix

SAINSBURYS
Chocolate Flavour Swiss Roll
Chocolate Orange Swiss Roll
Jam Vanilla Flavour Roll
Junior Chocolate with
    Buttercream Roll
Junior Jam Swiss Roll
Milk Chocolate Swiss Roll
Raspberry Flavour Swiss Roll

♦ = negligible

Grams per 25g/1oz (approx) | 1 2 3 4 5 6 7 8 9 10 11 12 13 14 15 16 17 18 19 20 21 22 23 24 25

Item	Grams per 25g/1oz (approx)
Super Swiss Roll with Blackcherry & Buttercream	
Super Swiss Roll with Strawberry Jam	
Super Swiss Roll with Apricot & Peach	
All Butter Walnut Sandwich	
Almond Slices	
Angel Cake	
Assorted Cup Cakes	
Battenburg Cake	
Cherry Bakewells	
Cherry & Coconut Sandwich	
Cherry Cake	
Choc Cup Cakes	
Choc & Mint Cup Cakes	
Choc Cake with Choc Flavoured Chips	
Chocolate Angel Cake	

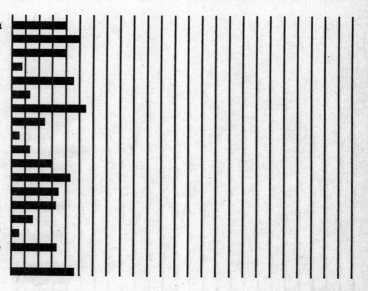

Chocolate Decorated Sandwich
Chocolate Delights
Coconut Cake
Coconut Crunch
Eccles Cakes
Family Size Genoa Cake
Flapjacks
Fondant Fancies
Fruity Malt Loaf
Ginger Cake
Iced Fruit Cake
Lemon Iced Cake
Madeira Cake
Spiced Fruit Cake
Sultana & Currant Cake
Wholemeal Honey & Fruit Loaf
Wholemeal Harvest Fruit Cake
Wholemeal Carrot & Orange
    Cake

♦ = negligible

Grams per 25g/1oz (approx)

Scale: 1 2 3 4 5 6 7 8 9 10 11 12 13 14 15 16 17 18 19 20 21 22 23 24 25

Tarts

Item	Grams per 25g/1oz (approx)
Apricot Pie	~4½
Bakewell Tart	~4
Blackcurrant Sundaes	~5½
Blackcurrant Pie	~4
Bramley Apple Pie	~4
Bramley Apple Crumbles	~4½
Deep Apple Pie	~4
Jam Tart	~4
Mince Pie	~4
Mincemeat Macaroons	~5½
Strawberry Sundaes	~5½
Treacle Tart	~4
Wholemeal Assorted Fruit Pie	~4½
Wholemeal Bramley Apple Pie	~4½

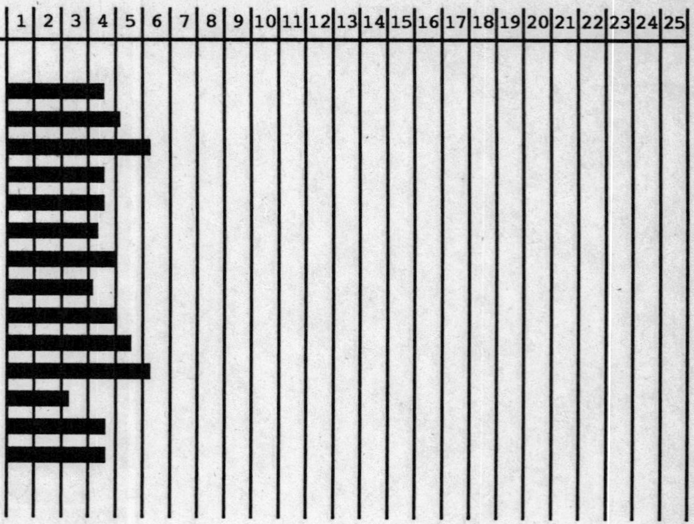

TESCO

67

Cream
Apple Fluted Sponge
Apricot Fluted Sponge
Chocolate Eclair
Fresh Cream Chocolate Sponge
    Bar
Fresh Cream Sponge Bar

Cake Decorations
Hundreds and Thousands
Jelly Diamonds
Orange & Lemon Slices
Sugar Strands, Assorted
Sugar Strands, Chocolate

Cake Mixes – Dry Mix
Batter
Chocolate Sponge Sandwich
Crumble
Luxury Chocolate Sponge
Luxury Sponge

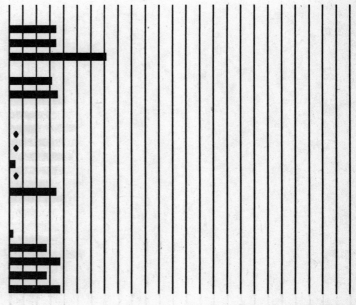

◆ = negligible

Grams per 25g/1oz (approx)	1	2	3	4	5	6	7	8	9	10	11	12	13	14	15	16	17	18	19	20	21	22	23	24	25

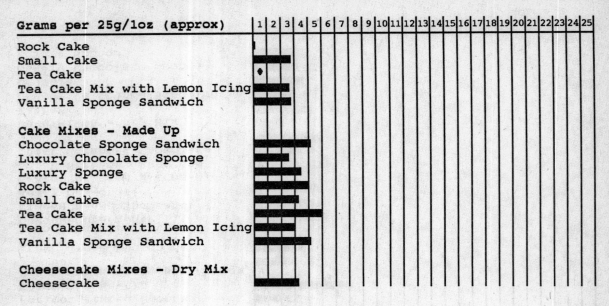

Rock Cake
Small Cake
Tea Cake
Tea Cake Mix with Lemon Icing
Vanilla Sponge Sandwich

Cake Mixes – Made Up
Chocolate Sponge Sandwich
Luxury Chocolate Sponge
Luxury Sponge
Rock Cake
Small Cake
Tea Cake
Tea Cake Mix with Lemon Icing
Vanilla Sponge Sandwich

Cheesecake Mixes – Dry Mix
Cheesecake

Chocolate Orange Flavour
    Crunch
Coffee Flavour Crunch
Luxury Strawberry Cheesecake
Luxury Tangerine Cheesecake
Lemon Meringue Crunch

Others
Almond Madeira with
    Buttercream Filling
Almond Rondo
Angel Cake
Apple, Jam and Nut Dessert
    Cake
Cherry Madeira
Corn Crisp
Dundee Cake
Flapjack
Fruits of the Forest Pies
Madeira Cake
Marble Cake

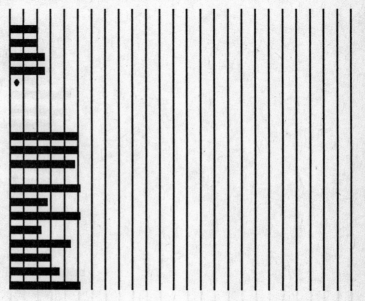

◆ = negligible

70

Grams per 25g/1oz (approx)	1 2 3 4 5 6 7 8 9 10 11 12 13 14 15 16 17 18 19 20 21 22 23 24 25
Meringue Flan	◆
Meringue Nests	◆
Rice Crisp	██████ (≈6)
Sponge Fingers	█ (≈1)
Sponge Flan Case	█ (≈1)
Trifle Sponge	█ (≈1)
Wholemeal Blackcurrant Pies	███ (≈3)
Wholemeal Fruit Cake	█▌ (≈1.5)
Swiss Roll	
Continental Apricot Jam & Hazelnut	████▌ (≈4.5)
Continental Chocolate	█████▌ (≈5.5)
Continental Strawberry	████ (≈4)
Deluxe Blackcurrant	███ (≈3)
Deluxe Chocolate	████▌ (≈4.5)
Deluxe Coffee & Hazelnut	████ (≈4)
Deluxe Strawberry	███ (≈3)

WAITROSE

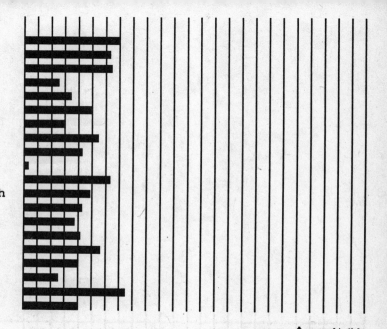

Frozen Shortcrust Pastry
Puff Pastry
Shortcrust Pastry
Battenberg
Mince Pies
Puff Pastry Mince Pies
Treacle Tarts
Chorley Cakes
Wholemeal Mince Pies
Trifle Sponge
Madeira/Buttercream
Lemon Iced Madeira Sandwich
Madeira Slice
All Butter Madeira Cake
All Butter Coconut Cake
Coconut Sandwich Cake
Iced Fruit Cake
Cherry Genoa
Walnut Layer Cake
Angel Cake

♦ = negligible

Grams per 25g/1oz (approx)

Food	1	2	3	4	5	6	7	8	9	10	11	12	13	14	15	16	17	18	19	20	21	22	23	24	25
Date & Walnut Cake	████
Light Fruit Cake	████
Whole Sultana Cake	███
Paradise Cake	█████
Rich Fruit Cake	████
Choc Gateau Roule Black Cherry	████
Choc Gateau Roule B'Cream	███████
Gateau Roule Black Cherry	█████
Gateau Roule Lemon Cheese	████
Gateau Roule Blackcurrant	████
Gateau Roule Strawberry	████
Milk Chocolate Rolls Raspberry	████
Milk Chocolate Rolls Vanilla	████████
Mini Rolls Strawberry	████
Summer Fruit Lattice Pie	█████
Tropical Fruit Lattice Pie	█████
Wholemeal Apple Mini Pies	█████

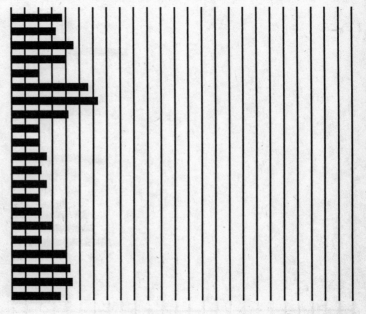

Wholemeal Blackcurrant Pies
Apple Pie
All Butter Eccles Cakes
Treacle Baked Roll
Sultana & Ginger Cake
Milk Chocolate Roll
Chocolate Sandwich
French Jam Sandwich
Original Plum Pudding
Round Christmas Pudding
Trad Christmas Pudding
Dundee Cake
Lux Rich Fruit - Marzipan
Christmas Cake
Lux Rich Fruit - Fully Iced
Iced Top Madeira Cake
Iced Rich Fruit Cake
Stollen with Marzipan
Frozen Chocolate Pavlova
Frozen Lemon Soufflé
Summer Fruit Russe

♦ = negligible

Grams per 25g/1oz (approx) — scale 1 to 25

Food	Grams per 25g/1oz (approx)
Frozen Choc Cream Gateau	5
Deluxe Strawberry Gateau	4
Deluxe Chocolate Gateau	4
Exotic Fruit Tart	3
Frozen Eclairs	7½
Frozen Profiteroles	6
Iced Danish Twists	6
Iced Buns with Jam	1
Iced Buns with Fruit	2
Sultana & Danish Pastry	5
Lemon Mousse Tart	7

CHEESE – GENERAL

Food	Grams per 25g/1oz (approx)
Diet Brie	3
Camembert	6
Cheddar	6
Diet White and Coloured Cheddar	4½
Mature Cheddar	8

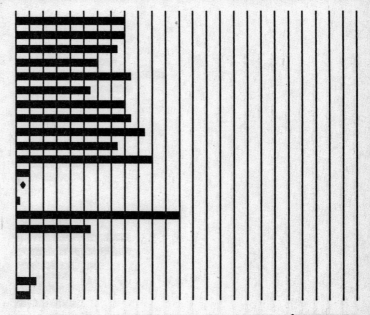

Vegetarian Cheddar
Cheshire
Danish Blue
Edam
Double Gloucester
Gouda
Gruyere
Red Leicester
Lymeswold
Parmesan
Stilton
Cottage with Cream
Cottage without Cream
Diet Cottage Cheese – Plain
Cream Cheese
Cheese Spread

BOOTS
Cottage Cheese – Cheddar &
    Onion
Cottage Cheese – Natural

◆ = negligible

Grams per 25g/1oz (approx)

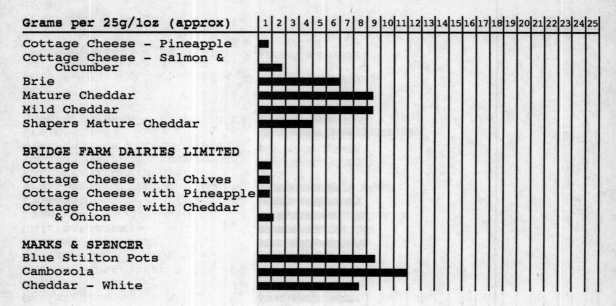

	1–25 scale
Cottage Cheese – Pineapple	~1
Cottage Cheese – Salmon & Cucumber	~2
Brie	~7
Mature Cheddar	~9
Mild Cheddar	~9
Shapers Mature Cheddar	~4
BRIDGE FARM DAIRIES LIMITED	
Cottage Cheese	~1
Cottage Cheese with Chives	~1
Cottage Cheese with Pineapple	~1
Cottage Cheese with Cheddar & Onion	~2
MARKS & SPENCER	
Blue Stilton Pots	~9
Cambozola	~12
Cheddar – White	~8

Cheddar - Red	
Cheddar - White Grated	
Cheddar Farmhouse Matured	
Cheddar Medium - Grated	
Cheddar with Onion & Chives	
Danish Blue	
Double Gloucester	
Doux de Montagne	
Edam	
Emmental	
Fresh Grated Parmesan Cheese	
Full Flav. Extra Mature Cheddar	
Gouda	
Gruyere	
Mature Cheddar - Fine Grated	
Medium Cheddar Cheese Slices	
Port Salut	
Roquefort	
Soft Cheese Spread with Butter	

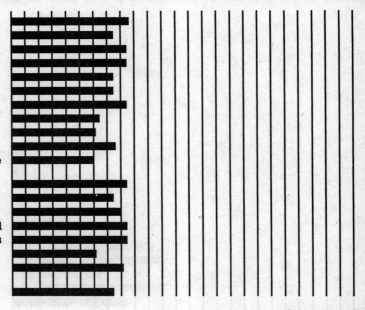

♦ = negligible

Grams per 25g/1oz (approx)	1	2	3	4	5	6	7	8	9	10	11	12	13	14	15	16	17	18	19	20	21	22	23	24	25
Stilton									▓																
Blue Brie											▓														
Brie							▓																		
Brie with Chives											▓														
Brie with Peppercorns										▓															
Cottage Cheese – Apple, Celery & Nut			▓																						
Cottage Cheese – Chicken & Asparagus			▓																						
Cottage Cheese – Tuna, Sweetcorn & Pepper		▓																							
Cottage Cheese Creamy – Prawns			▓																						
Cottage Cheese Creamy – Natural			▓																						
Cottage Cheese Snack – Prawn			▓																						
Cottage Cheese with Pineapple	▓																								
Cottage Cheese with Prawns			▓																						

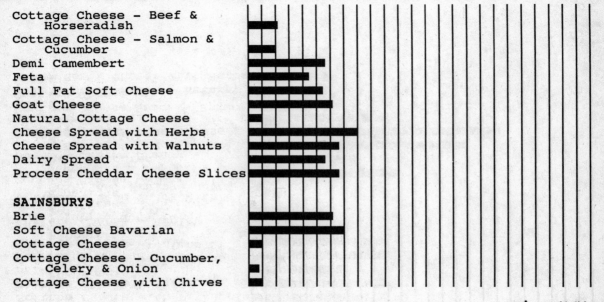

Cottage Cheese – Beef & Horseradish

Cottage Cheese – Salmon & Cucumber

Demi Camembert

Feta

Full Fat Soft Cheese

Goat Cheese

Natural Cottage Cheese

Cheese Spread with Herbs

Cheese Spread with Walnuts

Dairy Spread

Process Cheddar Cheese Slices

SAINSBURYS

Brie

Soft Cheese Bavarian

Cottage Cheese

Cottage Cheese – Cucumber, Celery & Onion

Cottage Cheese with Chives

◆ = negligible

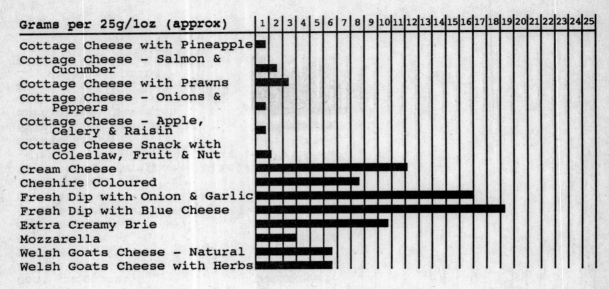

Grams per 25g/1oz (approx)

	1 2 3 4 5 6 7 8 9 10 11 12 13 14 15 16 17 18 19 20 21 22 23 24 25
Cottage Cheese with Pineapple	
Cottage Cheese - Salmon & Cucumber	
Cottage Cheese with Prawns	
Cottage Cheese - Onions & Peppers	
Cottage Cheese - Apple, Celery & Raisin	
Cottage Cheese Snack with Coleslaw, Fruit & Nut	
Cream Cheese	
Cheshire Coloured	
Fresh Dip with Onion & Garlic	
Fresh Dip with Blue Cheese	
Extra Creamy Brie	
Mozzarella	
Welsh Goats Cheese - Natural	
Welsh Goats Cheese with Herbs	

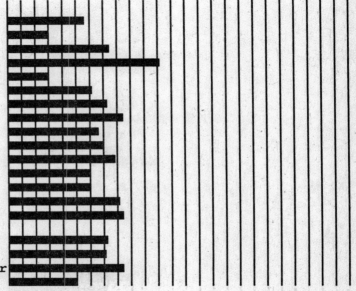

Welsh Goats Cheese with Sweet Peppers
Bavarian Blue Cheese
Creamery
Cream Cheese with Chives
Curd Cheese
Cheese Spread
Danish Blue
Danish Mycella
Dolcelatte
Doux de Montagne
Double Gloucester/Stilton
Edam
Edam Slices
English Cheddar Slices
Farmhouse Cheddar
Full Fat Soft Cheese with Garlic & Parsley
Gorgonzola
Grated English Mature Cheddar
Grated Mozzarella

♦ = negligible

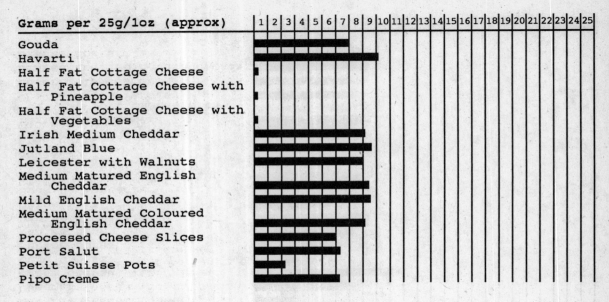

Grams per 25g/1oz (approx)	1	2	3	4	5	6	7	8	9	10	11	12	13	14	15	16	17	18	19	20	21	22	23	24	25
Gouda																									
Havarti																									
Half Fat Cottage Cheese																									
Half Fat Cottage Cheese with Pineapple																									
Half Fat Cottage Cheese with Vegetables																									
Irish Medium Cheddar																									
Jutland Blue																									
Leicester with Walnuts																									
Medium Matured English Cheddar																									
Mild English Cheddar																									
Medium Matured Coloured English Cheddar																									
Processed Cheese Slices																									
Port Salut																									
Petit Suisse Pots																									
Pipo Creme																									

Roquefort
Svenbo
Low Fat Cheese (Cheddar Type)
Low Fat Cheese (Edam Type)
Soft Bavarian with
    Horseradish
Skimmed Milk Soft Cheese
St Paulin
White Cheshire
Half Fat Creamery

ST IVEL

Cheese
Blue Stilton
Caerphilly
Cheddar
Cheshire
Double Gloucester
Lancashire
Leicester

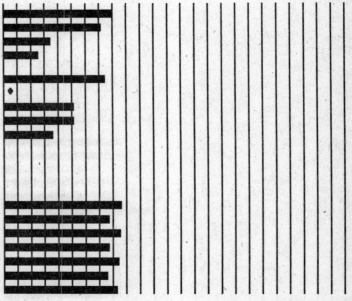

♦ = negligible

84

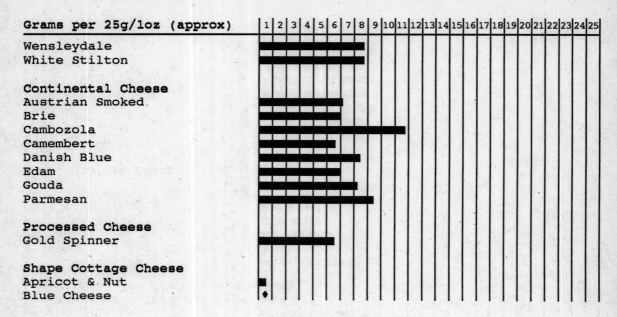

Grams per 25g/1oz (approx)	1	2	3	4	5	6	7	8	9	10	11	12	13	14	15	16	17	18	19	20	21	22	23	24	25
Wensleydale								8																	
White Stilton								8																	
Continental Cheese																									
Austrian Smoked						6																			
Brie						6																			
Cambozola											11														
Camembert						6																			
Danish Blue							7																		
Edam						6																			
Gouda							7																		
Parmesan								8																	
Processed Cheese																									
Gold Spinner						6																			
Shape Cottage Cheese																									
Apricot & Nut	1																								
Blue Cheese	1																								

85

Caribbean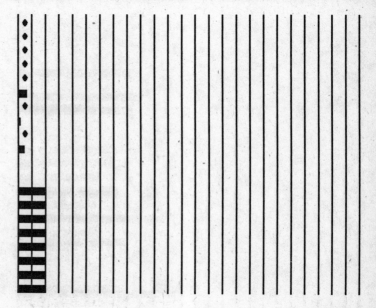
Italian Style
Mexican
Natural
Onion & Chives & Dill
Onion & Cheddar
Pineapple
Prawn & Cucumber
Smoked Cheese
Tuna & Cashew Nut

Shape Low Fat Cheese
Blue Cheese
Garlic & Herbs
Ham
Onion & Chives
Orange
Pineapple
Plain Soft Cheese
Walnut

◆ = negligible

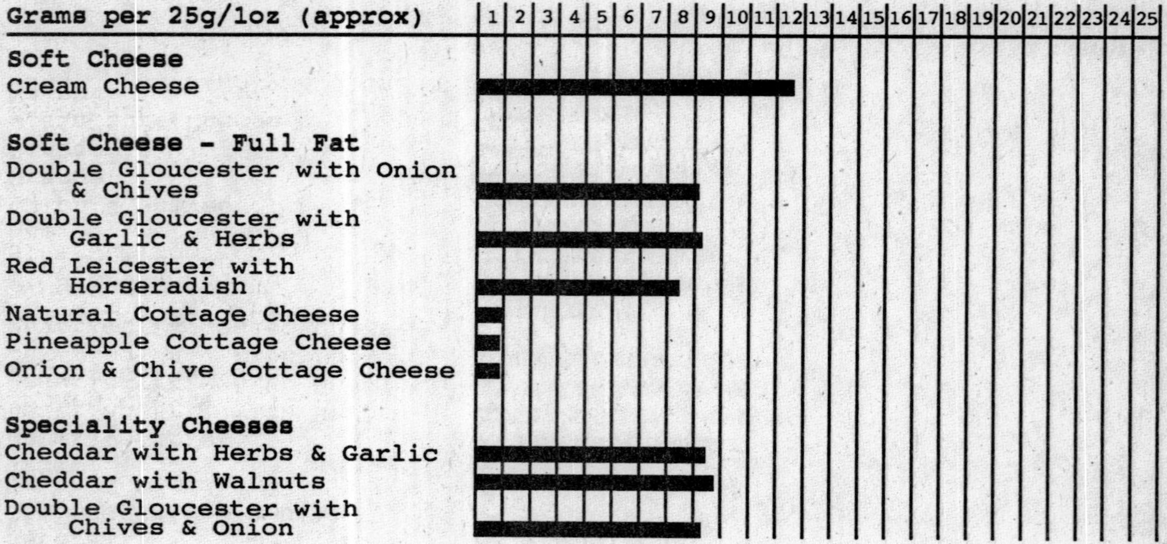

Grams per 25g/1oz (approx)

Scale: 1 to 25

Soft Cheese

Cheese	Grams per 25g/1oz (approx)
Cream Cheese	≈12

Soft Cheese – Full Fat

Cheese	Grams per 25g/1oz (approx)
Double Gloucester with Onion & Chives	≈9
Double Gloucester with Garlic & Herbs	≈9
Red Leicester with Horseradish	≈8
Natural Cottage Cheese	≈1
Pineapple Cottage Cheese	≈1
Onion & Chive Cottage Cheese	≈1

Speciality Cheeses

Cheese	Grams per 25g/1oz (approx)
Cheddar with Herbs & Garlic	≈9
Cheddar with Walnuts	≈10
Double Gloucester with Chives & Onion	≈9

Family Favourites
Pizza Style
Smoky Cheddar with Paprika &
    Onion
Vegetarian

TESCO
Bavarian Brie
Bavarian Brie with Herbs
Bavarian Brie with Mushrooms
Bavarian Brie with Peppers
Bavarian Processed Cheese,
    Ham & Pepper
Blue Creme Cheese
Blue Stilton
Brie
Brie Royale
Caerphilly
Cambozola
Camembert
Cheddar with Chives & Onion

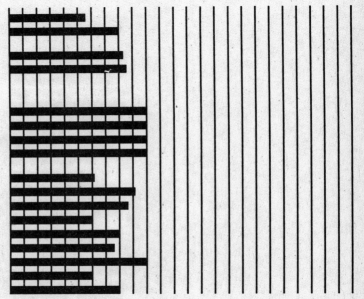

♦ = negligible

Grams per 25g/1oz (approx)	1	2	3	4	5	6	7	8	9	10	11	12	13	14	15	16	17	18	19	20	21	22	23	24	25
Cheddar with Pickle	████████																								
Cheddar with Port & Stilton	█████████																								
Cheddar, all types	█████████																								
Cheese & Onion Spread, Tub	██████																								
Cheese & Prawn Spread, Tub	██████																								
Cheese Spread Natural, Tub	██████																								
Cheese Spread, Swiss Gruyere	███████																								
Cheese Spread, Triangles	██████																								
Cheshire	████████																								
Chevre (Goats Milk Cheese)	███████																								
Curd Cheese with Walnut	███████																								
Danish Blue	█████████																								
Danish Blue Gold	██████████																								
Dolcelatte	█████████																								
Double Gloucester	█████████																								
Double Gloucester with Caerphilly & Onion	████████																								
Double Gloucester with Onion & Chives	████████																								

89

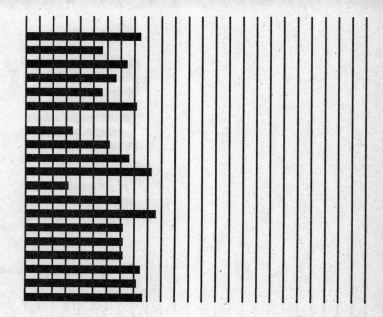

Double Gloucester with
    Stilton
Edam
Emmental
Gorgonzola
Gouda
Gruyere
Half Fat Cheese (Cheddar
    Type)
Jarlsberg
Lancashire
Lymeswold
Medium Fat Curd Cheese
Melbury
Mycella
Parmesan
Parmesan Wedge
Processed Cheese
Red Leicester
Red Leicester & Walnuts
Roule Herbs & Garlic

90

♦ = negligible

Grams per 25g/1oz (approx)

Cheese	Grams per 25g/1oz (approx)
Skimmed Milk Cheese	1
Soft Dairy Cheese with Pineapple	7
Soft Dairy Cheese with Chives	7
Soft Dairy Cheese, Plain	7
St Paulin	6
Swiss Gruyere Cheese Spread	7
Vegetarian Cheddar	8
Wensleydale	8
White Stilton	7

UNITED CO-OPERATIVE DAIRIES

Cheese	Grams per 25g/1oz (approx)
Leicester	8
Wensleydale	8
Lancashire	8
Caerphilly	8
Blue Stilton	8
Derby	8
Double Gloucester	8

Cheshire
Cheddar

WAITROSE
Home Produced Cheddar
Extra Mild Cheddar
English Cheddar
English Mature Cheddar
Red English Cheddar
Vegetarian Cheddar
Irish Cheddar
Farmhouse Cheddar
Australian Cheddar
Canadian Cheddar
Dutch Edam
Dutch Gouda
Edam Halves
Havarti
Danish Samsoe
Farmhouse Double Gloucester
Farmhouse Red Leicester

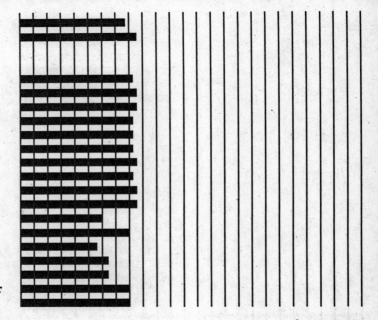

◆ = negligible

Grams per 25g/1oz (approx)

Cheese	Grams per 25g/1oz (approx)
Lancashire	8
Farmhouse Caerphilly	8
Wensleydale	8
Farmhouse Mature Mini Cheddar	9
Farmhouse Mini Double Glouc	8
Cottage Cheese	1
Cottage Cheese – Onion & Chives	1
Cottage Cheese – Chicken & Mushroom	1
Cottage Cheese – Onions & Cheddar	2
Cottage Cheese – Ham & Pineapple	1
Cottage Cheese with Prawns	1
Diet Cottage Cheese	0.5
Cream Cheese with Chives	12
Full Fat Soft Cheese	7
Curd Cheese	3

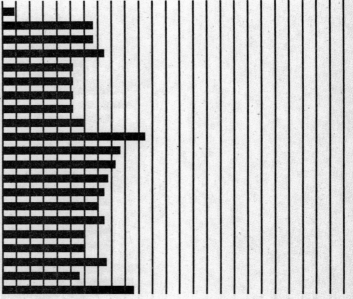

Cottage Cheese - Mixed Beans
Danish Blue Mild
Danish Blue Mature
Danish Blue Extra Mature
Cheese Spread
Cheddar Cheese Spread
Cheddar Cheese Spread - Prawn
Curd Cheese Spread
Somerset Brie Quarters
Cambozola
Blue Stilton
Farmhouse Mature Cheddar
White Stilton
Danish Blue
Dolcelatte
Emmentaler
Smoked Cheese
Smoked Cheese with Ham
French Brie Supreme
Camembert
German Brie with Mushroom

94

♦ = negligible

Grams per 25g/1oz (approx)	1	2	3	4	5	6	7	8	9	10	11	12	13	14	15	16	17	18	19	20	21	22	23	24	25
French Brie																									
German Brie																									
German Brie Blue																									
Double Gloucester – Chives & Onions																									
Sage Derby																									
White Cheshire																									
Red Cheshire																									
English Cheddar with Walnuts																									
Extra Mature Cheddar																									
Chevre Goat																									
Lys Bleu																									
Weekend Brie																									
Roule																									
Brie with Mixed Peppers																									
Brie with Herbs																									
Italian Parmesan																									
Bavarian Smoked Cheese																									
Jarlsberg																									

Swiss Gruyere
Esprom
Danbo
Red Vein Cheddar
Jarlsberg
Emmental
Mountain Gorgonzola
Tomme De Neige
Danish Samsoe
Tilsiter

CONDIMENTS - GENERAL
Apple Sauce
Bovril
Cranberry Sauce
Curry Powder
English Mustard
Ginger Ground
Horseradish Sauce
Marmite
Mustard Powder

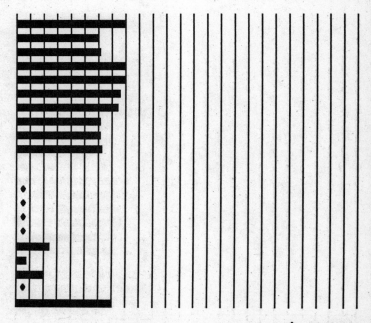

♦ = negligible

Grams per 25g/1oz (approx)	1	2	3	4	5	6	7	8	9	10	11	12	13	14	15	16	17	18	19	20	21	22	23	24	25
Oxo Cubes	▮																								
Pepper	▬																								
Redcurrant Jelly	◆																								
Sage & Onion Stuffing	▮																								
Salt	◆																								
Tartare Sauce	▬▬▬▬▬▬																								
Vinegar	◆																								
RHM GROCERY (PAXO & BISTO)																									
Sage & Onion Stuffing Mix	▮																								
Parsley & Thyme Stuffing Mix	▮																								
Apple & Herb Stuffing Mix	▮																								
Golden Breadcrumbs	▮																								
Bread Sauce Mix	▮																								
Bisto Powder	◆																								
Bisto Gravy Granules	▮																								
Bisto Gravy Granules for Chicken	▮																								
Bisto Cheese Sauce Granules	▮▮																								

Bisto Parsley Sauce Granules

SAINSBURY
Country Stuffing Mix
Sage & Onion Stuffing Mix

TESCO
Bramley Apple Sauce
Cranberry Sauce
English Mustard
Fresh Garden Mint
Horseradish Cream
Horseradish Sauce
Mint Jelly
Mint Sauce
Redcurrant Jelly
Sauce Tartare
Curry Powder
Ginger
Ground Black Pepper
Nutmeg

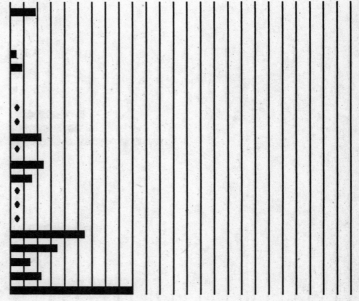

♦ = negligible

Grams per 25g/1oz (approx)	1	2	3	4	5	6	7	8	9	10	11	12	13	14	15	16	17	18	19	20	21	22	23	24	25
Table Salt	♦																								
Country Herb Stuffing																									
Parsley and Thyme Stuffing																									
Sage and Onion Stuffing																									
WAITROSE																									
Malt Vinegar	♦																								
Mint Sauce	♦																								
Sage & Onion Stuffing																									
Parsley & Thyme Stuffing																									
Country Herb Stuffing																									
Gravy Granules																									
Beef Cubes																									
Chicken Cubes																									
Beef Stock Drink	♦																								
Sea Salt – Coarse	♦																								
Sea Salt – Fine	♦																								
Table Salt	♦																								
Cooking Salt	♦																								

CONFECTIONERY - GENERAL

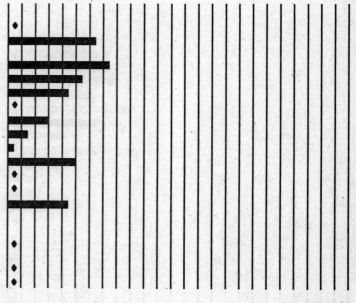

Boiled Sweets
Bounty Bar
Chocolate, Average, Milk or Plain
Chocolate - Nut & Raisin
Chocolate - Fancy & Filled
Fruit Gums
Fudge
Humbugs
Liquorice
Mars Bar
Pastilles
Peppermints
Toffees

BOOTS

Acid Drops
Assorted Chocolate Coated Almonds
Barley Sugar Drops

100

◆ = negligible

Grams per 25g/1oz (approx)	1	2	3	4	5	6	7	8	9	10	11	12	13	14	15	16	17	18	19	20	21	22	23	24	25
Butter Drops	▇																								
Mint Drops	•																								
Mint Drops Assortment	•																								
Mint Humbugs	▇																								
Mixed Fruit Flavour Drops	•																								
Olde Fashioned Drop Assortment	•																								
Ginger & Pear Bar	▇	▇	▇																						
Swiss Style Muesli Bar	▇	▇	▇																						
Date & Muesli Bar	▇	▇	▇																						
Fruit & Nut Bar with Honey	▇	▇	▇	▇	▇																				
CADBURYS																									
Apricot and Almond	▇	▇	▇	▇	▇	▇	▇	▇																	
Autumn Nuts	▇	▇	▇	▇	▇	▇	▇	▇	▇																
Biarritz	▇	▇	▇	▇	▇	▇	▇																		
Boost	▇	▇	▇	▇	▇	▇	▇	▇																	
Bournville	▇	▇	▇	▇	▇	▇	▇																		
Buttons	▇	▇	▇	▇	▇	▇	▇	▇																	

Caramel
Caramel Bunnies
Caramels
Chocolate Cream
Chocolate Eclairs
Contrast
Creme Eggs
Crunchie
Curly Wurly
Dairy Milk
Double Decker
Five Centre
Flake
Fruit and Nut
Fruit Bonbons
Fudge
Ginger
Go
Golden Crisp
Grande Seville
Hazel in Caramel

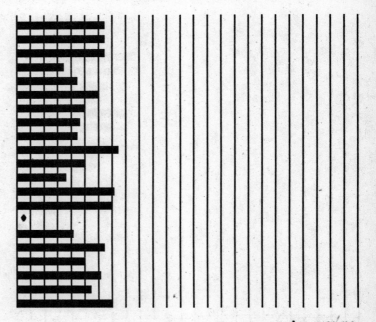

♦ = negligible

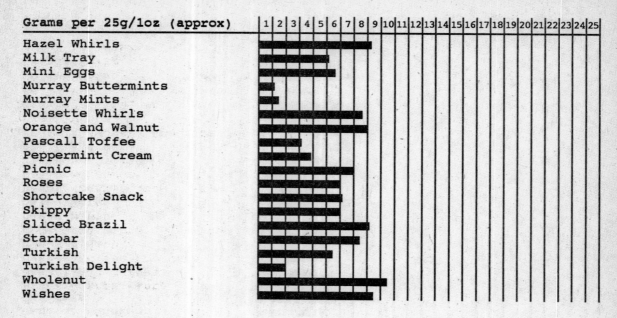

Wispa

CO-OP
After Dinner Mints
Brazil Nut Toffee
Butter Toffee Pop Corn
Chewy Fruits
Chocolate Mints
Clear Mints
Dairy Fudge
Devon Cream Toffee
Dolly Mixtures
Fruit Pastilles
Fruit Flavoured Pastilles
Fruit Flavoured Assortment
Fruit Drops
Fruit Jellies
Jelly Bears
Jelly Beans
Jelly Babies
Jolly Jellies

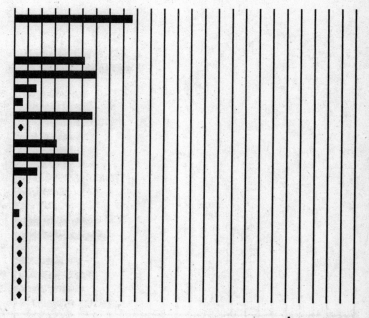

◆ = negligible

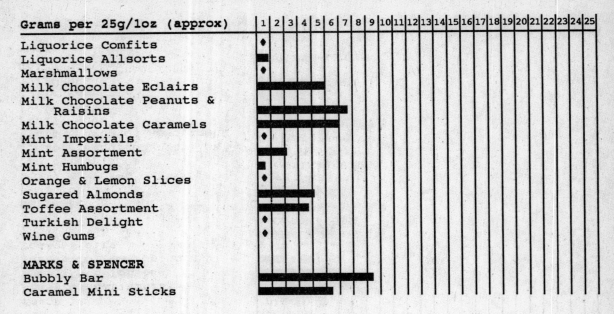

Chunky Milk Chocolate
Crunch
Fudge Bars
Hazelnut Mini Sticks
Honeycomb Crunch
Jet Peanut Bar
Milk Choc with Strawberry &
    Cream
Milk Chocolate
Milk Chocolate with Hazelnuts
Milk Chocolate Mini Sticks
Mini Stick Gift Pack
Mocca Mini Sticks
Assorted Mini Sticks
Plain Chocolate
Strawberry Creme Bar
After Dinner Mints
Chocolate Ginger
Doyens
Fresh Cream Chocolate
    Truffles

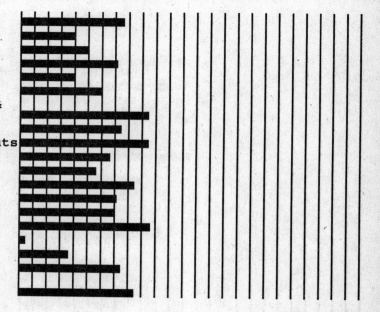

106

♦ = negligible

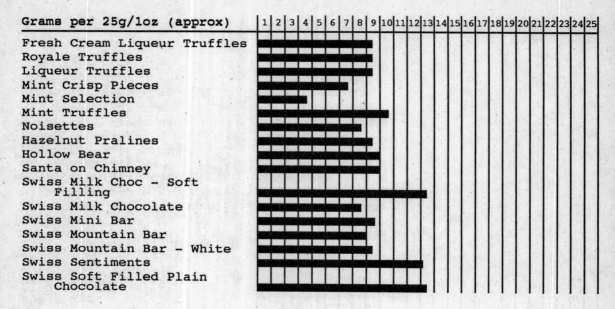

Grams per 25g/1oz (approx)	Grams
Fresh Cream Liqueur Truffles	9
Royale Truffles	9
Liqueur Truffles	9
Mint Crisp Pieces	7
Mint Selection	4
Mint Truffles	10
Noisettes	8
Hazelnut Pralines	9
Hollow Bear	9
Santa on Chimney	9
Swiss Milk Choc – Soft Filling	13
Swiss Milk Chocolate	8
Swiss Mini Bar	9
Swiss Mountain Bar	9
Swiss Mountain Bar – White	9
Swiss Sentiments	12
Swiss Soft Filled Plain Chocolate	13

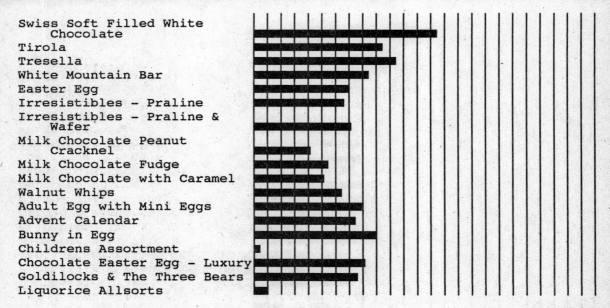

Swiss Soft Filled White Chocolate	
Tirola	
Tresella	
White Mountain Bar	
Easter Egg	
Irresistibles – Praline	
Irresistibles – Praline & Wafer	
Milk Chocolate Peanut Cracknel	
Milk Chocolate Fudge	
Milk Chocolate with Caramel	
Walnut Whips	
Adult Egg with Mini Eggs	
Advent Calendar	
Bunny in Egg	
Childrens Assortment	
Chocolate Easter Egg – Luxury	
Goldilocks & The Three Bears	
Liquorice Allsorts	

♦ = negligible

Grams per 25g/1oz (approx)

Product	1	2	3	4	5	6	7	8	9	10	11	12	13	14	15	16	17	18	19	20	21	22	23	24	25
Luxury Assortment							▇																		
Luxury Assortment – Penny Bazaar							▇																		
Plain/Milk Chocs Fruit & Nut				▇																					
Apple Cream Filled Bar						▇																			
Assorted Mini Sticks								▇																	
Milk Chocolate Birds Eggs			▇																						
Milk Chocolate Buttons							▇																		
Milk Chocolate Drops			▇																						
Nest Egg								▇																	
Rabbit & Hare								▇																	
Spring is Sprung								▇																	
Springtime Madness								▇																	
White Chocolate Buttons							▇																		
Fruit Chews	▇																								
Fruit Pastilles	◆																								
Liquorice Sandwiches	▇																								
Real Fruit Gums	◆																								
Real Fruit Jellies	◆																								

109

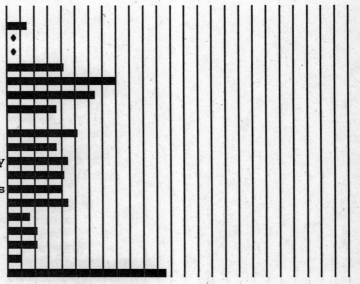

Sherbet Fruit Flavoured
    Assortment
Soft Gum Animals
Wine Gums
Assorted Liqueurs
Champagne Truffles
Cocktail Chocolates
Cointreau Sticks
Luxury Milk Chocolate
    Liqueurs
Marzipan Fruits
Mini Gifts – Cointreau/Sherry
Mini Gifts – Liqueurs
Muscatel de Valencia Liqueurs
Bitter Chocolate Mints
Butter Mintos
Buttermints
Chocolate Mints
Mint Assortment
Almond Clusters

♦ = negligible

110

Grams per 25g/1oz (approx)

Product	1	2	3	4	5	6	7	8	9	10	11	12	13	14	15	16	17	18	19	20	21	22	23	24	25
Milk & White Chocolate Peanuts								8																	
Mini Gifts – Almonds									9																
Mini Gifts – Hazelnuts											11														
Sugared Almonds						6																			
Butter Toffee Assortment					5																				
Milk Chocolate Caramels/Fudge					5																				
Milk Chocolate Eclairs					5																				
Milk/Plain Choc – Caramel Centre					5																				
Soft & Smooth Caramels					5																				
Vanilla Toffee							7																		
Butter Fudge, Trad					5																				
Milk & White Chocolate Raisins			3																						
Spanish Almonds & Honey Crunch								8																	

111

NESTLE
Animal Bar
Dairy Crunch
White Dairy Crunch
Fruit & Nut
Milk
Milky Bar
Milky Bar Buttons
Plain Superfine
Raisin & Biscuit
Superfruit & Nut
Chocolate Praline
Dark Praline
Chocolate Truffle
Mocca Truffle
Chocolate Yes Cake
Caramel Yes Cake

SAINSBURYS
Acid Drops
American Hard Gums

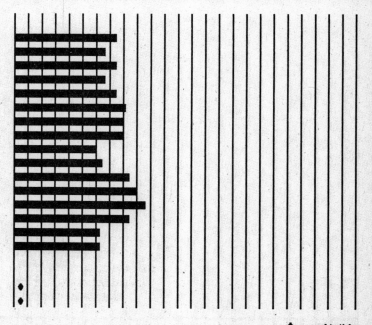

♦ = negligible

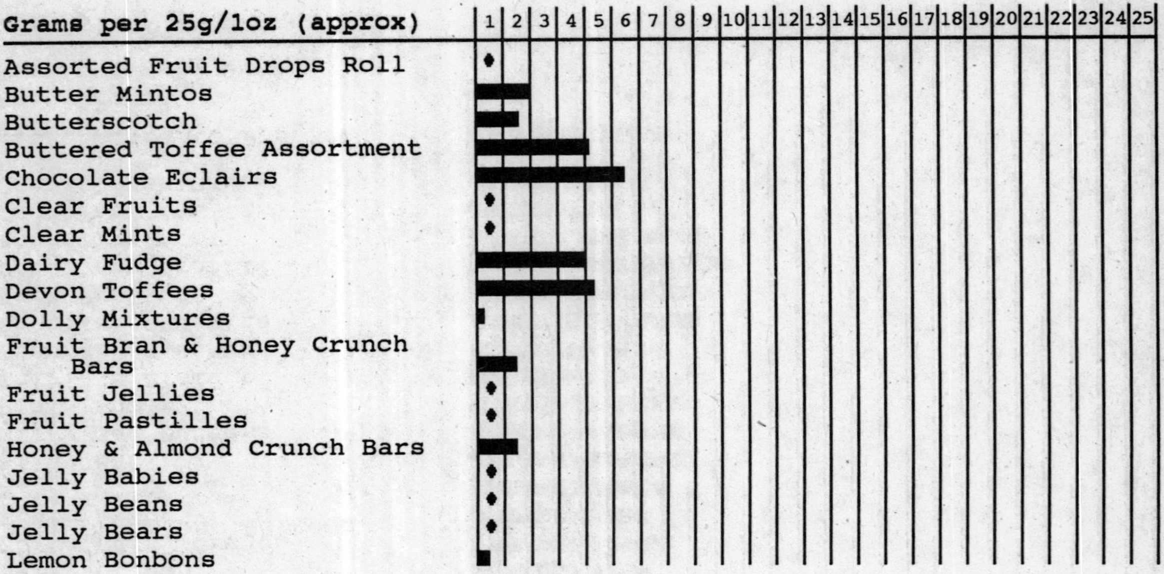

Grams per 25g/1oz (approx)

	1	2	3	4	5	6	7	8	9	10	11	12	13	14	15	16	17	18	19	20	21	22	23	24	25

Assorted Fruit Drops Roll
Butter Mintos
Butterscotch
Buttered Toffee Assortment
Chocolate Eclairs
Clear Fruits
Clear Mints
Dairy Fudge
Devon Toffees
Dolly Mixtures
Fruit Bran & Honey Crunch
    Bars
Fruit Jellies
Fruit Pastilles
Honey & Almond Crunch Bars
Jelly Babies
Jelly Beans
Jelly Bears
Lemon Bonbons

113

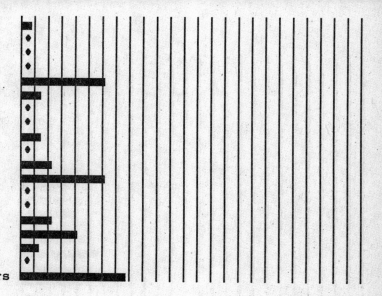

Liquorice Allsorts
Liquorice Comfits
Liquorice Catherine Wheels
Marshmallows
Milk Chocolate Buttons
Mini Allsorts
Mini Jellies
Mini Wine Gums
Mint Humbugs
Mint Imperials
Mint Lumps
Peanut Brittle
Sherbet Cocktail
Soft Mints
Toffee Bonbons
Toffee Nut Puffs
Toffee Popcorn
Wine Gums
Milk Chocolate Fun Time Bars

◆ = negligible

Grams per 25g/1oz (approx)	1	2	3	4	5	6	7	8	9	10	11	12	13	14	15	16	17	18	19	20	21	22	23	24	25

TESCO

Product	Grams per 25g/1oz (approx)
American Hard Gums	◆
Brazil Nut Toffee	5
Childrens Pack	1
Chocolate Nut and Raisins	6
Cream Toffees	5
Dolly Mixtures	1
Fruit Jellies	◆
Fruit Pastilles	◆
Fudge	4
Jelly Babies	◆
Jelly Beans	◆
Liquorice Allsorts	1
Liquorice Catherine Wheels	◆
Liquorice Comfits	◆
Liquorice Twists	◆
Marshmallows	◆
Mini Allsorts	2
Mini Wine Gums	◆

Mint Humbugs	
Mint Imperials	
Sparkling Fruits	
Sparkling Mints	
Sugar Letters	
Wine Gums	
WAITROSE	
Devon Toffee	
Mint Assortment	
Butter Mintos	
Clear Mints	
Mint Humbugs	
Mint Imperials	
Dairy Fudge	
Jelly Babies	
Fruit Pastilles	
Liquorice Allsorts	
Wine Gums	
Chocolate Eclairs	
Soft Nougat	

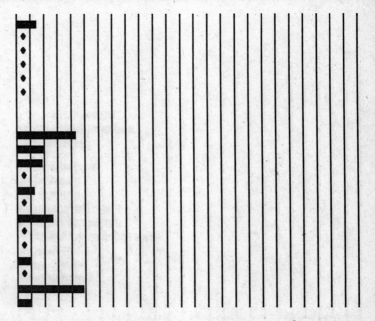

♦ = negligible

116

Grams per 25g/1oz (approx)

Confectionery	Grams per 25g/1oz (approx)
Clear Fruits	◆ (≈1)
Fruit Jellies	◆ (≈1)
Dairy Toffees	≈5
Chocolate Mint Crisp	≈5
Chocolate Ginger	≈3
Chocolate Brazils	≈11
White Chocolate	≈7½
White Chocolate & Nuts	≈7½
Chocolate Bar with Mint Fill	≈5
Chocolate Bar with Strawberry	≈5
Milk Chocolate with Caramel	≈6
Milk Chocolate with Coffee Cream	≈6
Plain Choc with Hazelnut	≈9
Plain Chocolate	≈7
Mint Creams	≈3

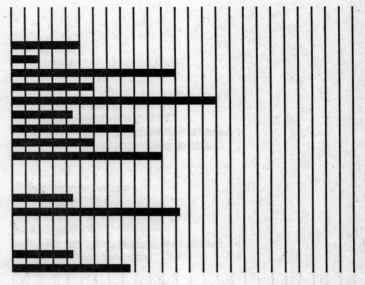

CREAM & CREAM SUBSTITUTES - GENERAL
Cream, Single
Shape, Single
Cream, Double
Shape, Double
Cream, Cornish Clotted
Cream, Soured
Cream, Whipping
Cream, Sterilised Canned
Dream Topping

NESTLE (Chambourcy)
Single Cream
Double Cream

SAINSBURYS
Single Cream - UHT
Canned Cream - Sterilised

118

♦ = negligible

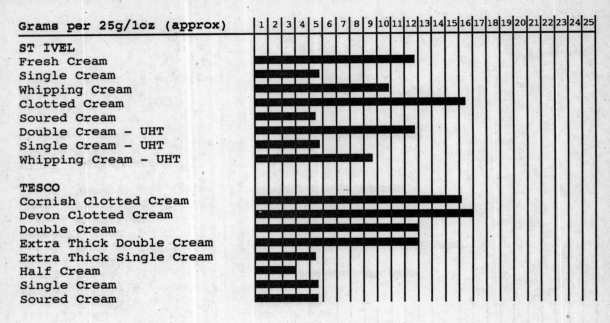

Grams per 25g/1oz (approx)	1	2	3	4	5	6	7	8	9	10	11	12	13	14	15	16	17	18	19	20	21	22	23	24	25

ST IVEL
Fresh Cream
Single Cream
Whipping Cream
Clotted Cream
Soured Cream
Double Cream – UHT
Single Cream – UHT
Whipping Cream – UHT

TESCO
Cornish Clotted Cream
Devon Clotted Cream
Double Cream
Extra Thick Double Cream
Extra Thick Single Cream
Half Cream
Single Cream
Soured Cream

119

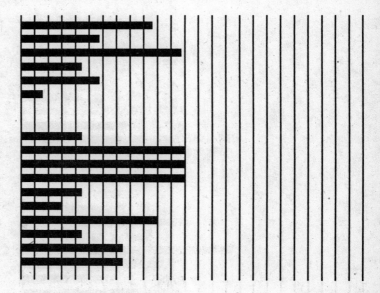

Whipping Cream
Sterilised - Canned
Longlife Double Cream
Longlife Single Cream
Double Cream Substitute
Single Cream Substitute

WAITROSE
Single Cream
Double Cream
Extra Thick Double Cream
Fresh Double Cream
Fresh Single Cream
Half Cream
Whipping Cream
Soured Cream
Spooning Cream
Brandy Cream

120

♦ = negligible

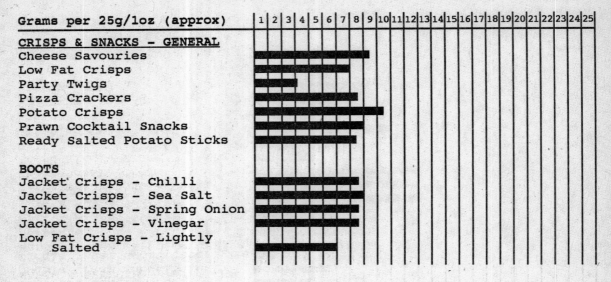

Grams per 25g/1oz (approx)	1	2	3	4	5	6	7	8	9	10	11	12	13	14	15	16	17	18	19	20	21	22	23	24	25

CRISPS & SNACKS - GENERAL

	Grams per 25g/1oz
Cheese Savouries	9
Low Fat Crisps	7
Party Twigs	3
Pizza Crackers	7
Potato Crisps	10
Prawn Cocktail Snacks	8
Ready Salted Potato Sticks	7

BOOTS

	Grams per 25g/1oz
Jacket Crisps - Chilli	8
Jacket Crisps - Sea Salt	8
Jacket Crisps - Spring Onion	8
Jacket Crisps - Vinegar	7
Low Fat Crisps - Lightly Salted	5

KP CRISPS
Standard Crisps
Lower Fat Crisps

MARKS & SPENCER
Assorted Multipack Crisps
Barbecue Beef & Onion Crisps
Barbecue Spare Rib Crisps
Chargrill Beef Crisps
Cheese & Onion Crisps
Cocktail Crisps
Corn Crisps – Californian
Crinkles – Lightly Salted
Crisps Beef Lower Fat
Crisps Cheese & Onion Lower
    Fat
Crisps Ready Salted Lower Fat
Homestyle Crisps
Lattice Crisps
Lightly Salted Low Fat Crisps
Lower Fat Crisp Assortment

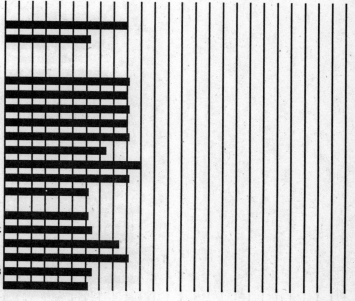

♦ = negligible

Grams per 25g/1oz (approx)

Food	Grams per 25g/1oz (approx)
Natural Salt & Vinegar Crisps	7
Ready Salted Crisps	9
Salt & Vinegar Crisps	10
Sour Cream & Chives Crisps	10
Spring Onion Crisps	10
Thick & Crunchy Crisps	10
Unsalted Crisps	9
Burger Bites	9
Cheese Savouries	8
Deltas	8
Indonesian Style Crackers	7
Mixed Pepper Flavour Chips	9
Mushroom/Garlic Flavour Crisps	8
Onion Flavour Chips	9
Pizza Bits – Italian Style	6
Potato Rings	7
Potato Squares	7
Potato Waffles	7

Prawn Cocktail Snacks
Prawn Crackers
Ready Salted Potato Sticks
Salt & Vinegar Chiplets
Scamps
Tortilla Chips

SAINSBURYS
Jacket Crisps – Malt Vinegar
Brontosaurus Ribs
Flintstone Snacks – Faces
Flintstone Snacks – Boulders
Bacon Crispies
Bacon Flavour Wholewheat
    Crisps
Cheesy Buttons
Cheese Flavour Puffs
Cheese & Ham Nibbles
Cheese Flavour Snacks
Cheese & Onion Crisps
Cheesy Nik Naks

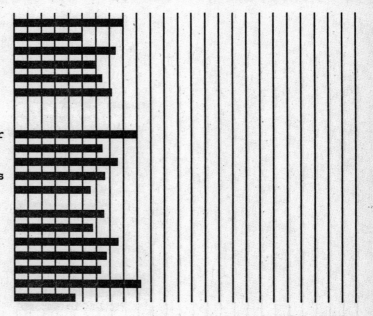

◆ = negligible

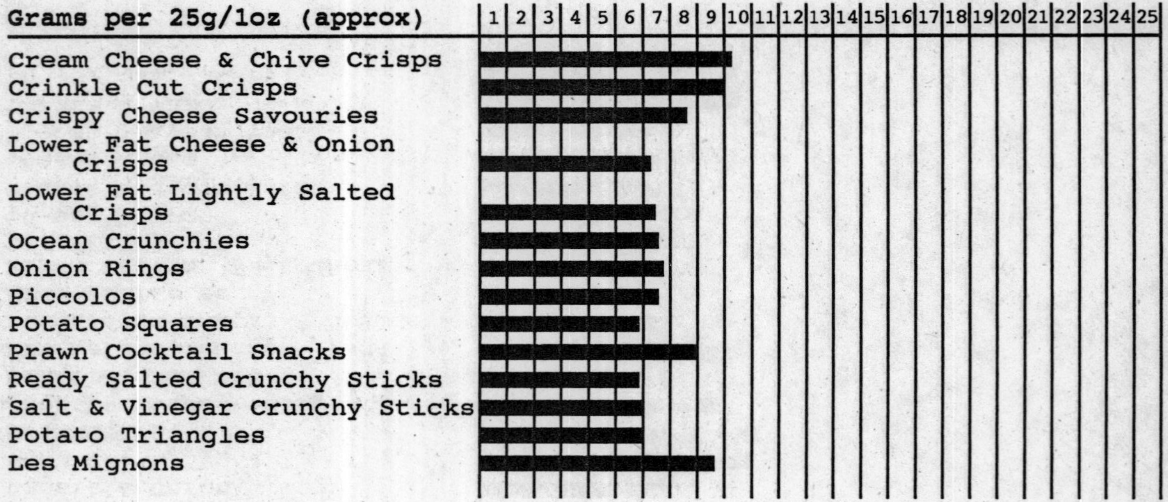

Grams per 25g/1oz (approx)

Food	Grams per 25g/1oz (approx)
Cream Cheese & Chive Crisps	9.5
Crinkle Cut Crisps	9.5
Crispy Cheese Savouries	8
Lower Fat Cheese & Onion Crisps	7
Lower Fat Lightly Salted Crisps	7.5
Ocean Crunchies	7.5
Onion Rings	7.5
Piccolos	7
Potato Squares	7
Prawn Cocktail Snacks	8
Ready Salted Crunchy Sticks	7
Salt & Vinegar Crunchy Sticks	7
Potato Triangles	7
Les Mignons	9

125

TESCO

Bacon Bites	
Beef Crisps	
Butterkist Butter Toffee Popcorn	
Cheese & Onion Crisps	
Corn Curls	
Crinkle Cut Crisps	
Crunchy Sticks Ready Salted	
Crunchy Sticks Salt & Vinegar	
Curry Crisps	
Lower Fat Crisps	
Onion Rings	
Potato Chips (Salt & Vinegar)	
Potato Chips Ready Salted	
Potato Rings	
Potato Triangles	
Prawn Cocktail Crisps	
Prawn Cocktail Snacks	
Ready Salted Crisps	
Salt & Vinegar Crisps	

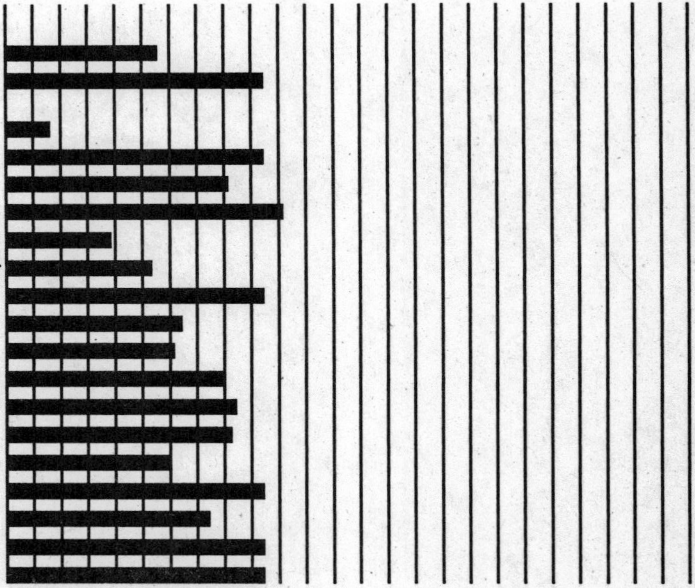

◆ = negligible

Grams per 25g/1oz (approx)	Amount
Spring Onion Crisps	~10
Tortilla Chips	~6.5
WAITROSE	
Crispy Thins	~6
Cheese Savouries	~8
Party Twigs	~3
Cheese Twists	~7
Peanut Sticks	~5
Caramel Peanut Popcorn	~4.5
Chocolate Mint Popcorn	~3
Chocolate Popcorn	~3
Salt & Vinegar Savoury Sticks	~6
Salt & Vinegar Potato Twirls	~5
Onion Rings	~6.5
Savoury Puffs	~11
Bacon Snacks	~5.5
Crinkle Crisps	~9
Ready Salted Crisps	~8.5

Salt & Vinegar Crisps
Cheese & Onion Crisps
Bouquet Garni Crisps
Sour Cream & Chives Crisps
Potato Sticks
Potato Rings
Prawn Cocktail Snacks
Lower Fat SP Onion Crisps
Lower Fat S&V Crisps
Lower Fat Unsalted Crisps

DELICATESSEN

SAINSBURYS
Carrot & Nut Slice
Houmous
Taramasalata
Tzatziki

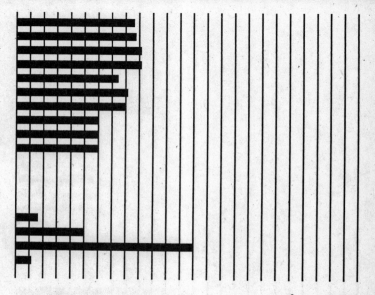

◆ = negligible

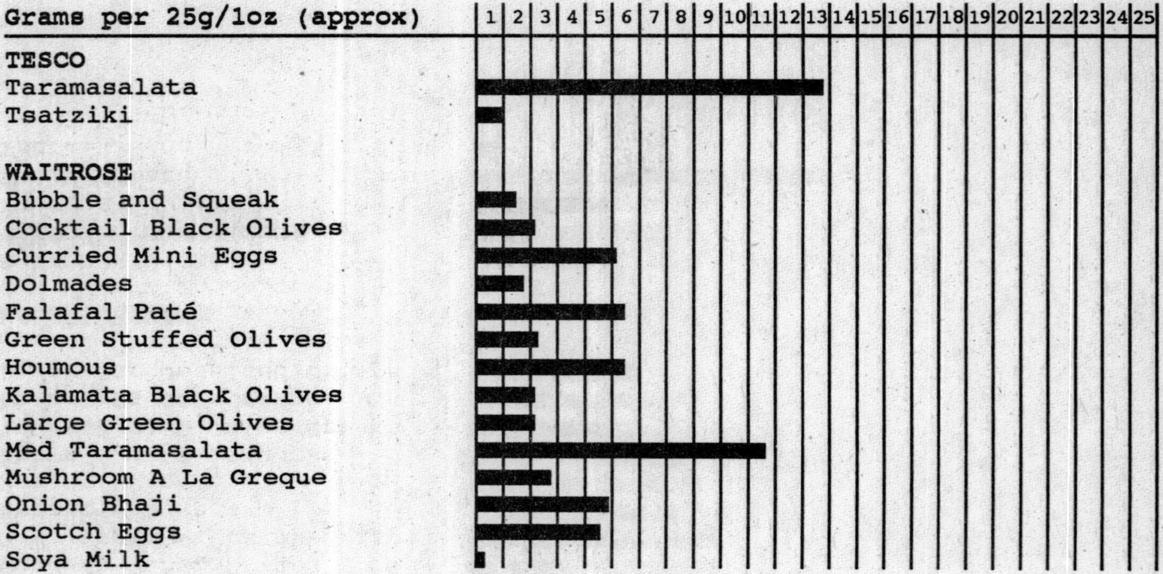

Grams per 25g/1oz (approx)	1	2	3	4	5	6	7	8	9	10	11	12	13	14	15	16	17	18	19	20	21	22	23	24	25

TESCO
Taramasalata
Tsatziki

WAITROSE
Bubble and Squeak
Cocktail Black Olives
Curried Mini Eggs
Dolmades
Falafal Paté
Green Stuffed Olives
Houmous
Kalamata Black Olives
Large Green Olives
Med Taramasalata
Mushroom A La Greque
Onion Bhaji
Scotch Eggs
Soya Milk

Tahinosalata
Taramasalata
Vegetable Pate

DIABETIC FOODS

BOOTS
Bourbon Cream Biscuits
Chocolate Coated Biscuits
Ginger Cream Biscuits
Lincoln Biscuits
Sandwich Wafer - Lemon
Cake Mix - Chocolate
Cake Mix - Plain
Milk Chocolate/Coffee
White Chocolate
Whole Lemon Drink
Whole Orange Juice
Apricot Jam
Blackcurrant Jam
Fine Cut Marmalade

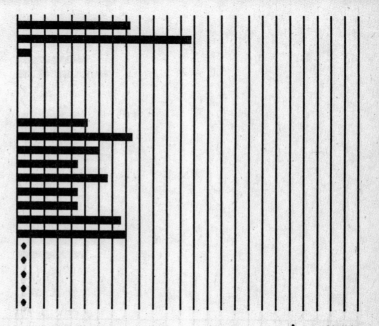

◆ = negligible

Grams per 25g/1oz (approx)

Item	1	2	3	4	5	6	7	8	9	10	11	12	13	14	15	16	17	18	19	20	21	22	23	24	25
Raspberry Jam	◆																								
Strawberry Jam	◆																								
Thick Cut Marmalade	◆																								
Plain Chocolate with Peppermint Filling	▓	▓	▓	▓	▓	▓																			
Milk Chocolate – Fruit & Nut	▓	▓	▓	▓	▓	▓	▓	▓	▓																
Milk Chocolate – Hazelnut	▓	▓	▓	▓	▓	▓	▓	▓																	
Milk Chocolate – Orange	▓	▓	▓	▓	▓	▓	▓	▓																	
Milk Chocolate – Peppermint	▓	▓	▓	▓	▓	▓	▓	▓																	
Milk Chocolate Bar	▓	▓	▓	▓	▓	▓	▓																		
Milk Chocolate Drops	▓	▓	▓	▓	▓	▓	▓																		
Plain Chocolate Bar	▓	▓	▓	▓	▓	▓	▓																		
Chocolate Chip Cookies	▓	▓	▓	▓	▓	▓																			
Country Cookies	▓	▓	▓	▓	▓																				
Fresh Mints	◆																								
Fruit Flavoured Drops	◆																								
Lemon Barley Drink	◆																								
Sandwich Chocolate Wafer	▓	▓	▓	▓	▓	▓	▓																		
Traditional Cookies	▓	▓	▓	▓	▓	▓																			

131

Lemonade	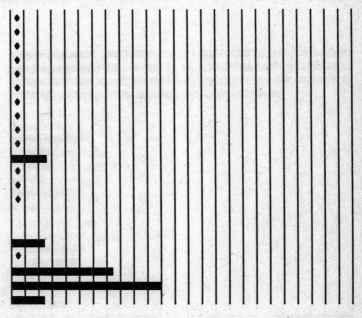	
Apricot Halves		
Fruit Cocktail		
Pear Quarters		
Sliced Peaches		
Jelly Crystals - Lemon		
Jelly Crystals - Orange		
Jelly Crystals - Raspberry		
Jelly Crystals - Strawberry		
Honey Spread		
Salad Dressing		
Blackcurrant Drink		
Blackcurrant Pastilles		
Fruit Flavoured Pastilles		

EGGS - GENERAL

Whole, Raw
White Only
Yolk Only
Dried
Boiled

◆ = negligible

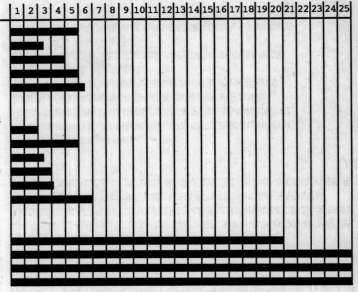

Grams per 25g/1oz (approx) — scale 1 to 25

Food	Grams per 25g/1oz (approx)
Fried	5
Poached	3
Omelette	4
Scotch Egg	5
Scrambled	6

EGG, CHEESE DISHES - GENERAL

Food	Grams per 25g/1oz (approx)
Cauliflower Cheese	2
Cheese Soufflé	2
Macaroni Cheese	3
Pizza, Cheese and Tomato	3
Quiche	4
Welsh Rarebit	6

FATS & OILS - GENERAL

Food	Grams per 25g/1oz (approx)
Butter	21
Coconut Oil	25
Cod Liver Oil	25
Compound Cooking Fat	25

Dripping, Beef
Flora
Gold Lowest
Lard
Low Fat Spread (e.g. Gold)
Margarine, all kinds
Olive Oil
Suet, Block
Suet, Shredded
Vegetable Oils

MARKS & SPENCER
Brandy Butter
Cornish Butter
English Butter Roll
English Churn
Golden Spread
Lite Low Fat Spread
Sunflower Margarine
Sunglow
Unsalted Butter

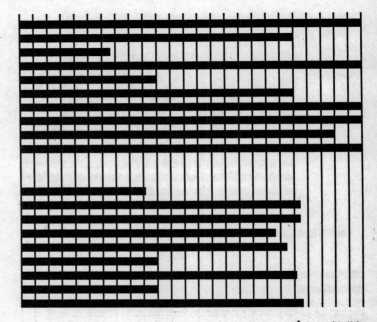

♦ = negligible

Grams per 25g/1oz (approx)

Product	Grams per 25g/1oz (approx)
Extra Virgin Olive Oil	25
Hazelnut Oil	25
Walnut Oil	25
SAINSBURYS	
Concentrated Butter	24
Blended Butter	21
Cornish Butter	21
English Butter	21
Continental Taste Butter	21
Somerset Butter Roll	21
Dutch Unsalted Butter	22
Continental Taste English Unsalted Butter	21
Normandy Butter	22
Luxury Soft Margarine	21
Margarine	21
Low Fat Spread	10
Soft Margarine	21

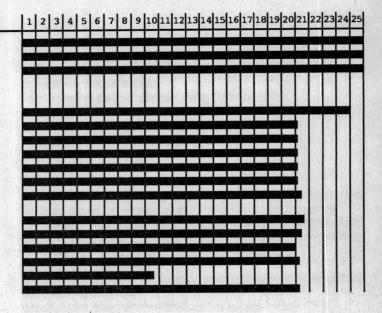

Soya Margarine
Sunflower Margarine
Pure Lard
Solid Vegetable Oil
Shorteen
Corn Oil
Extra Virgin Olive Oil
Groundnut Oil
Olive Oil
Sunflower Oil
Soya Oil
Vegetable Oil
Low Fat Sunflower Spread
Golden Low Fat
Devon Spread

TESCO
Margarine - Sunflower
Margarine - Premier
Margarine - Supersoft
Margarine - Soft

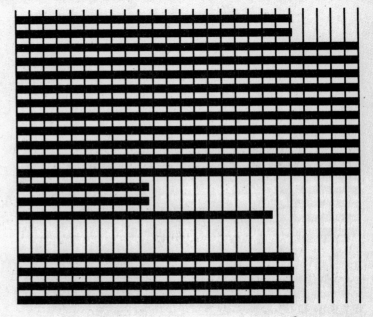

♦ = negligible

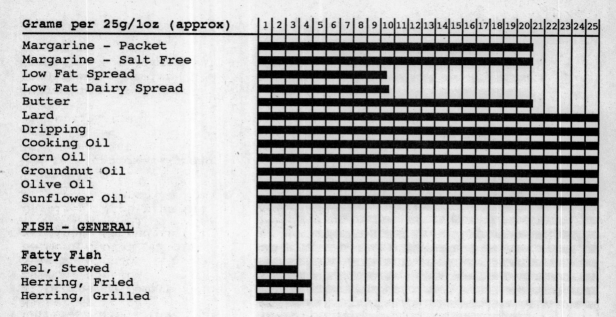

Grams per 25g/1oz (approx)	1	2	3	4	5	6	7	8	9	10	11	12	13	14	15	16	17	18	19	20	21	22	23	24	25

Margarine - Packet
Margarine - Salt Free
Low Fat Spread
Low Fat Dairy Spread
Butter
Lard
Dripping
Cooking Oil
Corn Oil
Groundnut Oil
Olive Oil
Sunflower Oil

FISH - GENERAL

Fatty Fish
Eel, Stewed
Herring, Fried
Herring, Grilled

137

Bloater, Grilled	
Kipper, Baked	
Mackerel, Fried	
Pilchards in Tomato Sauce	
Salmon, Steamed	
Salmon, Canned	
Salmon, Smoked	
Sardines, Canned in Oil (fish only)	
Sardines, Fish plus Oil	
Sardines, Canned in Tomato Sauce	
Sprats, Fried with Bones	
Trout (Brown), Steamed with Bones	
Tuna	
Whitebait, Fried	
White Fish	
Cod, Baked	
Cod, Fried in Batter	

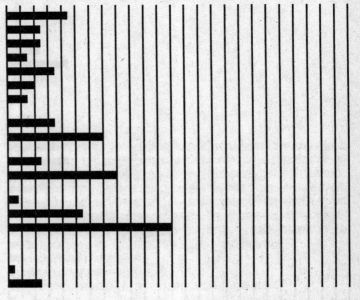

♦ = negligible

Grams per 25g/1oz (approx)	1	2	3	4	5	6	7	8	9	10	11	12	13	14	15	16	17	18	19	20	21	22	23	24	25
Cod, Grilled	▓																								
Cod, Poached	▓																								
Cod, Steamed	▓																								
Cod, Smoked, Poached	▓																								
Haddock, Fried	▓▓																								
Haddock, Steamed	▓																								
Haddock, Smoked, Steamed	▓																								
Halibut, Steamed	▓																								
Lemon Sole, Fried	▓▓																								
Lemon Sole, Steamed	▓																								
Plaice, Fried in Batter	▓▓▓▓																								
Plaice, Fried in Breadcrumbs	▓▓▓																								
Plaice, Steamed	▓																								
Whiting, Fried	▓▓																								
Whiting, Steamed	▓																								

Other Seafood

	1	2	3	4	5	6	7	8	9	10	11	12	13	14	15	16	17	18	19	20	21	22	23	24	25
Dogfish, Fried in Batter	▓▓▓▓																								
Skate, Fried in Batter	▓▓																								

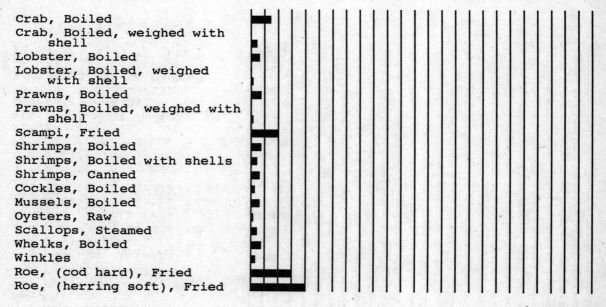

Crab, Boiled	
Crab, Boiled, weighed with shell	
Lobster, Boiled	
Lobster, Boiled, weighed with shell	
Prawns, Boiled	
Prawns, Boiled, weighed with shell	
Scampi, Fried	
Shrimps, Boiled	
Shrimps, Boiled with shells	
Shrimps, Canned	
Cockles, Boiled	
Mussels, Boiled	
Oysters, Raw	
Scallops, Steamed	
Whelks, Boiled	
Winkles	
Roe, (cod hard), Fried	
Roe, (herring soft), Fried	

♦ = negligible

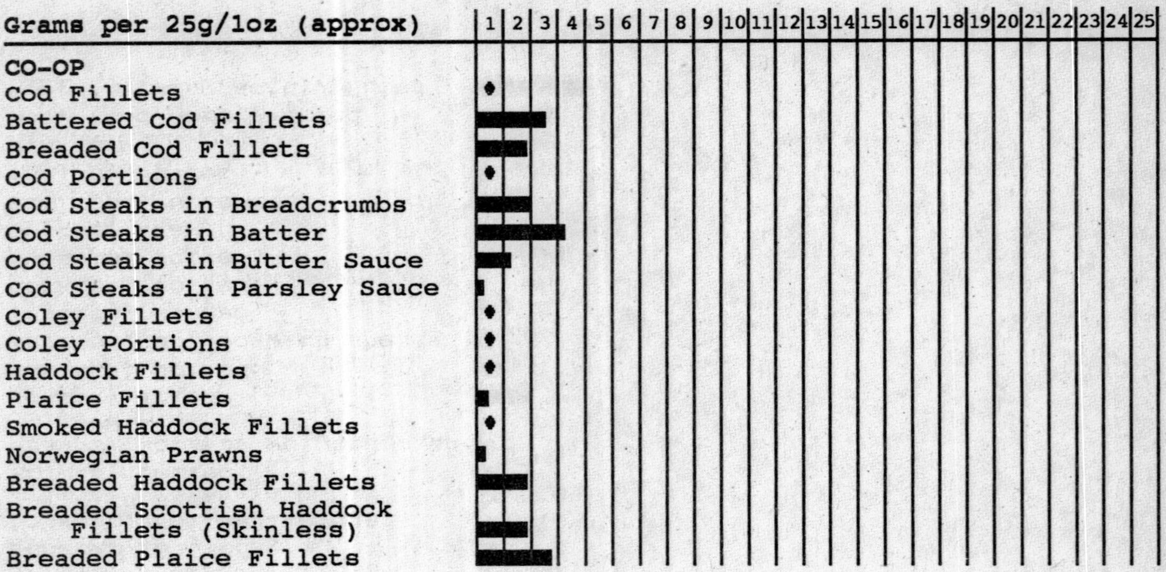

Grams per 25g/1oz (approx)	1	2	3	4	5	6	7	8	9	10	11	12	13	14	15	16	17	18	19	20	21	22	23	24	25

CO-OP

Horizontal bar chart of grams per 25g/1oz (approx):

- Cod Fillets — ~1
- Battered Cod Fillets — ~3
- Breaded Cod Fillets — ~2.5
- Cod Portions — ~1
- Cod Steaks in Breadcrumbs — ~2.5
- Cod Steaks in Batter — ~3.5
- Cod Steaks in Butter Sauce — ~1.5
- Cod Steaks in Parsley Sauce — ~1
- Coley Fillets — ~1
- Coley Portions — ~1
- Haddock Fillets — ~1
- Plaice Fillets — ~1
- Smoked Haddock Fillets — ~1
- Norwegian Prawns — ~1
- Breaded Haddock Fillets — ~2.5
- Breaded Scottish Haddock Fillets (Skinless) — ~2
- Breaded Plaice Fillets — ~3

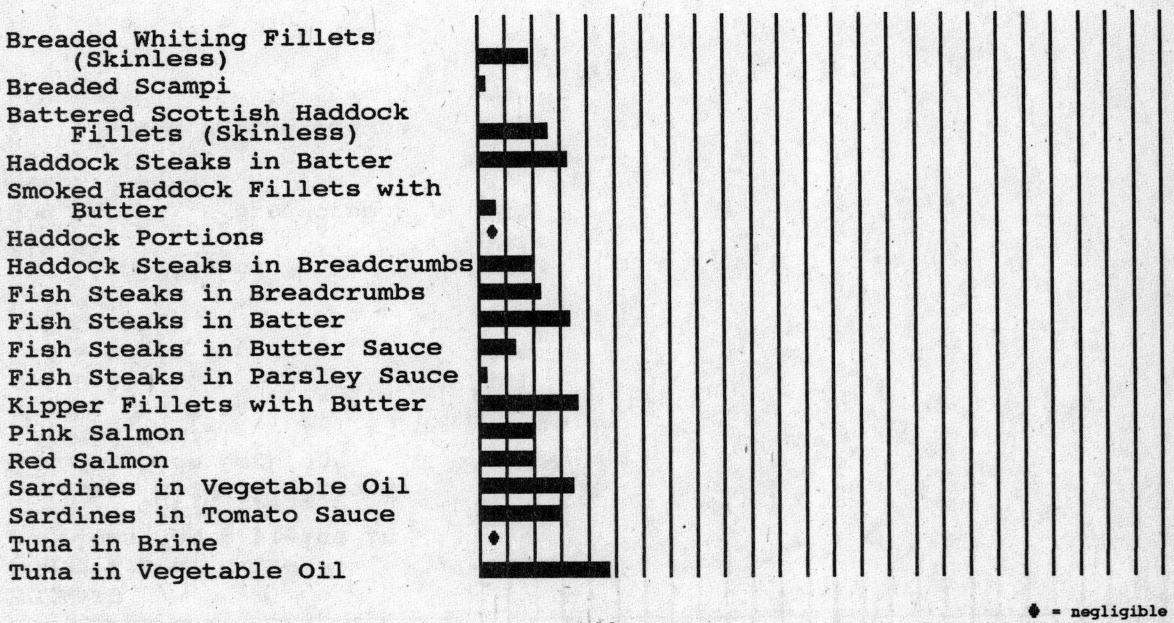

Breaded Whiting Fillets (Skinless)	
Breaded Scampi	
Battered Scottish Haddock Fillets (Skinless)	
Haddock Steaks in Batter	
Smoked Haddock Fillets with Butter	
Haddock Portions	
Haddock Steaks in Breadcrumbs	
Fish Steaks in Breadcrumbs	
Fish Steaks in Batter	
Fish Steaks in Butter Sauce	
Fish Steaks in Parsley Sauce	
Kipper Fillets with Butter	
Pink Salmon	
Red Salmon	
Sardines in Vegetable Oil	
Sardines in Tomato Sauce	
Tuna in Brine	
Tuna in Vegetable Oil	

♦ = negligible

142

Grams per 25g/1oz (approx)	1	2	3	4	5	6	7	8	9	10	11	12	13	14	15	16	17	18	19	20	21	22	23	24	25

ICELAND

	1	2	3	4	5	6	7	8	9	10	11	12	13	14	15	16	17	18	19	20	21	22	23	24	25
Boned Kipper Cutlets	██████																								
Boneless Whole Plaice in Breadcrumbs	██████																								
Boneless Haddock Fillets	████																								
Breaded Fish Portions																									
Breaded Scampi	●																								
Chunky Cod Bites	██████																								
Cod Bake	████																								
Cod & Chips for Two	█████																								
Cod Crumble	█																								
Cod Fillets	█																								
Cod Fish Fingers	████																								
Cod Kiev	█████																								
Cod Steaks in Breadcrumbs	████																								
Coley Steaks	●																								
Coley Fillets	●																								
Extra Large Peeled Prawns	█																								

143

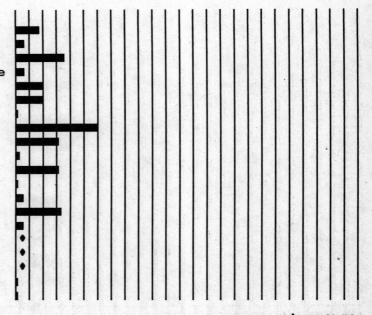

Fish Portions in Crispy Breadcrumbs	
Fish Steaks in Butter Sauce	
Fish & Cheese Grills	
Fish Steaks in Parsley Sauce	
Haddock Steaks	
Haddock Cordon Bleu	
Haddock Fillets	
Hot Smoked Mackerel Fillets	
Kipper Fillets	
Lemon Sole Fillets	
Lemon Sole Kiev	
North Atlantic Prawns	
Ocean Pie	
Oven Bake Plaice Fillets	
Plaice Fillets	
Skinless Cod Fillets	
Skinless Haddock Fillets	
Smoked Haddock Cutlets	
Smoked Haddock Fillets	
Whiting Fillets	

♦ = negligible

Grams per 25g/1oz (approx)	1	2	3	4	5	6	7	8	9	10	11	12	13	14	15	16	17	18	19	20	21	22	23	24	25
Whole Rainbow Trout		▓																							
MARKS & SPENCER																									
Bakeable Fish & Chips				▓																					
Cod Fillets in Breadcrumbs	▏																								
Cod Fish Cakes		▓																							
Cod in Light Ovencrisp Batter Frozen		▓																							
Fish Fingers			▓																						
Haddock Fillets Breaded	▏																								
Haddock Fillets Crispy Breadcrumbs	▏																								
Haddock Kiev				▓																					
Haddock Oven Crispy Batter Frozen				▓																					
Haddock in Light Ovencrisp Batter Frozen		▓																							
Lemon Sole Goujons					▓																				
Lemon Sole in Breadcrumbs	▏																								

Plaice Goujons
Plaice in Breadcrumbs Frozen
Plaice in Ovencrisp Crumb
Salmon Fishcakes
Scottish Cod Fillets in
    Ovencrisp Crumb
Scottish Cod in Ovencrisp
    Batter Frozen
Scottish Haddock Ovencrisp
    Crumb Frozen
Scottish Whiting Ovencrisp
    Crumb
Scottish Smoked Salmon
Smoked Mackerel Fillets
Smoked Rainbow Trout
Crab Paté
Smoked Mackerel Paté
Smoked Salmon Paté
Cod & Prawn Pie
Cod & Ratatouille Gratin

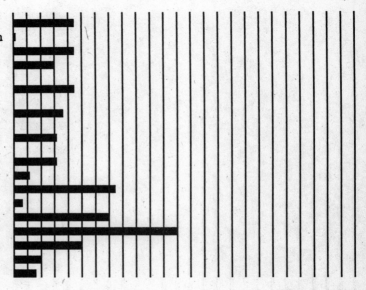

◆ = negligible

Grams per 25g/1oz (approx)	1	2	3	4	5	6	7	8	9	10	11	12	13	14	15	16	17	18	19	20	21	22	23	24	25
Cod Fillets – Cheese & Tomato Topping	██																								
Cod Florentine	██																								
Cod Linguine	█▌																								
Cod Pie – Pastry Topped	◆																								
Cod in Butter Sauce	█▌																								
Cod in Parsley Sauce	█▌																								
Crowns of Plaice	██																								
Dumplings	██																								
Fish Crumble	██																								
Fishermans Pie	███																								
Haddock & Vegetable Pie	█▌																								
Haddock Fillets – Herb Topping	███																								
Haddock Mornay	██																								
Haddock & Courgette Bake	██																								
Lobster Thermidor	██▌																								
Mariners Bake	██																								
Mediterranean Style Fish Soup	█																								

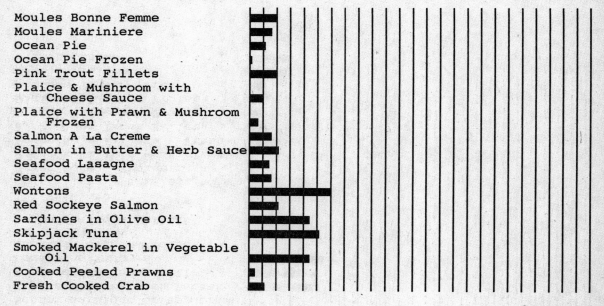

Moules Bonne Femme
Moules Mariniere
Ocean Pie
Ocean Pie Frozen
Pink Trout Fillets
Plaice & Mushroom with
    Cheese Sauce
Plaice with Prawn & Mushroom
    Frozen
Salmon A La Creme
Salmon in Butter & Herb Sauce
Seafood Lasagne
Seafood Pasta
Wontons
Red Sockeye Salmon
Sardines in Olive Oil
Skipjack Tuna
Smoked Mackerel in Vegetable
    Oil
Cooked Peeled Prawns
Fresh Cooked Crab

♦ = negligible

Grams per 25g/1oz (approx)

Item	Grams per 25g/1oz (approx)
Scampi in Light Crispy Crumb	<1
Kipper Fillets with Butter	5
Kippered Mackerel Fillets	5
Loch Fyne Kippers	6
Scottish Golden Haddock Cutlet	<1
Smoked Haddock Fillets	<1
Cod Fillets – Chunky, Skinless	<1
Cod Fillets – Skinless	<1
Dover Sole – Frozen	<1
Haddock Fillets – Skinless	<1
Lemon Sole Fillets – Fresh	1
Pink Flesh Trout Fillets	3
Plaice Fillets – Fresh	1
Plaice Fillets – Frozen	1
Rainbow Trout – Fresh	1
Salmon Fillets	3
Salmon Steaks	3

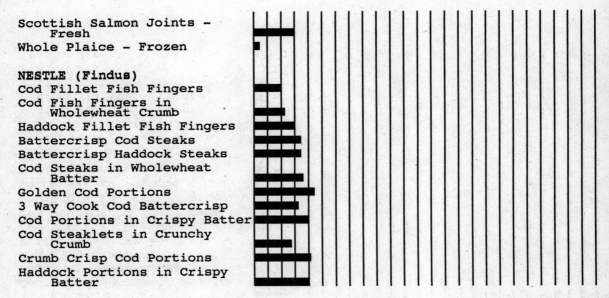

Scottish Salmon Joints – Fresh

Whole Plaice – Frozen

NESTLE (Findus)

Cod Fillet Fish Fingers

Cod Fish Fingers in Wholewheat Crumb

Haddock Fillet Fish Fingers

Battercrisp Cod Steaks

Battercrisp Haddock Steaks

Cod Steaks in Wholewheat Batter

Golden Cod Portions

3 Way Cook Cod Battercrisp

Cod Portions in Crispy Batter

Cod Steaklets in Crunchy Crumb

Crumb Crisp Cod Portions

Haddock Portions in Crispy Batter

♦ = negligible

150

Grams per 25g/1oz (approx)	1	2	3	4	5	6	7	8	9	10	11	12	13	14	15	16	17	18	19	20	21	22	23	24	25
Haddock Steaklets in Crunchy Crumb																									
Crumb Crisp Haddock Portions																									
Whole Breaded Plaice																									
Cod Fish Cakes																									
Plaice Fish Cakes																									
Cod Steak in Butter Sauce																									
Cod Steak in Cheese Sauce																									
Cod Steak in Parsley Sauce																									
Cod Steak in Seafood Sauce																									
Cod a L'Orange																									
Cod Au Gratin																									
Cod Bonne Femme																									
Cod Florentine																									
Cod Jardiniere																									
Cod Provencale																									
Haddock Parisienne																									

SAINSBURYS

Fish - Coated

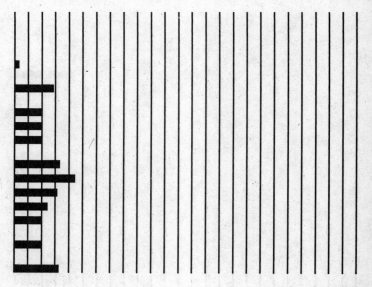

Chunky Cod Fillets

Cod Fillets in Golden
    Breadcrumbs

Skinless Cod Fillets in
    Natural Crispy Crumb

Cod Medallions

Cod Nuggets

Cod Oven Steaks in Crispy
    Batter

Cod in Light Crispy Batter

Fish Cakes

Cod Fillet Fish Fingers

Minced Cod Fish Fingers

Skinless Haddock Fillets in
    Natural Crispy Crumb

Haddock Steaks in Natural
    Crispy Crumb

◆ = negligible

Grams per 25g/1oz (approx)	1	2	3	4	5	6	7	8	9	10	11	12	13	14	15	16	17	18	19	20	21	22	23	24	25
Haddock in Light Crispy Batter	███																								
Haddock Fillets in Crispy Batter	█																								
Haddock Steaks in Crispy Batter	█																								
Oven Fish & Chips	██																								
Lemon Sole Fillets in Natural Crispy Crumb	██																								
Fish – Frozen																									
Cod Fillets	◆																								
Prime Skinless Cod Fillets	◆																								
Coley Fillets	◆																								
Haddock Cutlets with Butter (boil in bag)	█																								
Haddock Fillets	▏																								
Smoked Haddock Fillets	▏																								
Boned Kippers with Butter	███																								

153

Whole Kippers
Lemon Sole Fillets
Plaice Fillets
Rainbow Trout – Grilled
Shetland Whiting Fillets

Fish – Canned
Anchovy Fillets in Oil
Mackerel Fillets in Brine
Mackerel Fillets in Oil
Mackerel Fillets in Tomato
    Sauce
Mackerel in Tomato Sauce
Mackerel in Brine
Pink Salmon
Red Salmon
Tuna in Brine
Southsea Tuna in Brine
Southsea Tuna in Soya Oil
Skipjack Tuna In Water
Skipjack Tuna in Soya Oil

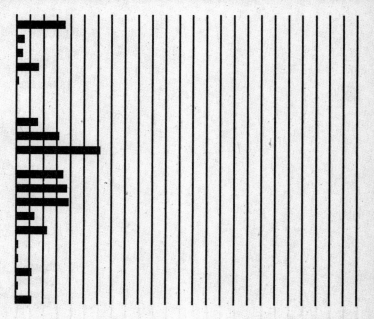

154

♦ = negligible

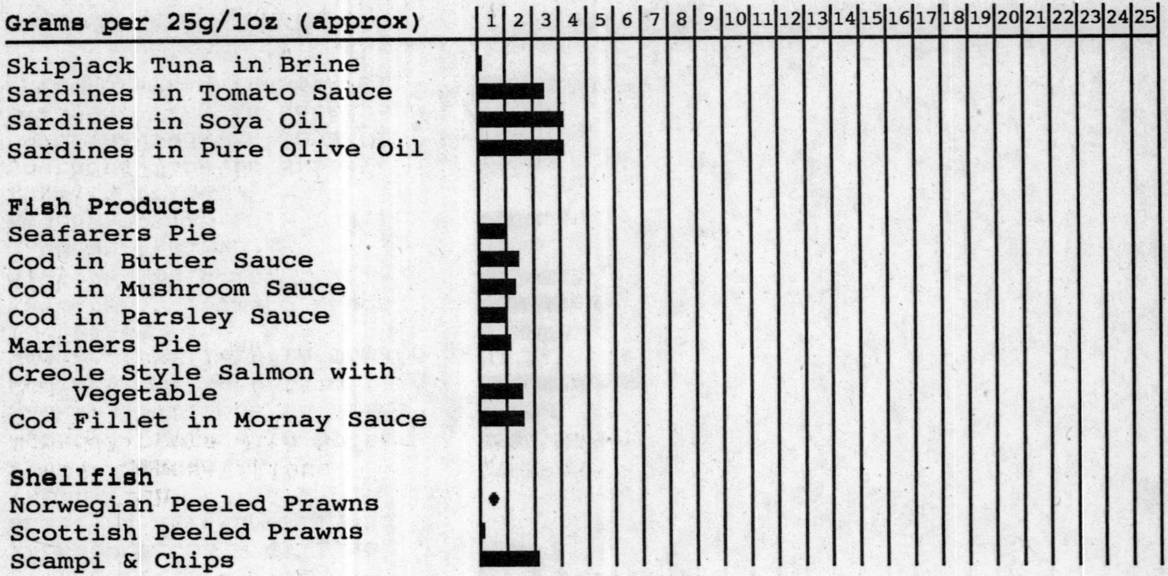

Grams per 25g/1oz (approx) 1 2 3 4 5 6 7 8 9 10 11 12 13 14 15 16 17 18 19 20 21 22 23 24 25

Skipjack Tuna in Brine
Sardines in Tomato Sauce
Sardines in Soya Oil
Sardines in Pure Olive Oil

Fish Products
Seafarers Pie
Cod in Butter Sauce
Cod in Mushroom Sauce
Cod in Parsley Sauce
Mariners Pie
Creole Style Salmon with
    Vegetable
Cod Fillet in Mornay Sauce

Shellfish
Norwegian Peeled Prawns
Scottish Peeled Prawns
Scampi & Chips

Breaded Scampi
Seafood Platter

TESCO

Fresh Fish
Boned Kipper Fillets
Boned Kippers with Butter
Cod Fillets
Cod Fillets in Batter
Cod Fillets in Breadcrumbs
Dover Sole
Eel
Grey Mullet
Haddock Fillets
Haddock Fillets in Batter
Haddock Fillets in
    Breadcrumbs
Haddock Goujons
Halibut
Herbed Smoked Mackerel

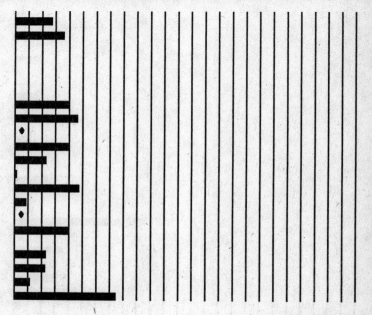

♦ = negligible

Grams per 25g/1oz (approx)	1	2	3	4	5	6	7	8	9	10	11	12	13	14	15	16	17	18	19	20	21	22	23	24	25
Herring Roe																									
Herrings																									
Kippers																									
Lemon Sole Fillets																									
Lobster - Brown Meat																									
Lobster - White Meat																									
Moules Au Gratin																									
Pink Trout Fillets																									
Plaice Fillets																									
Plaice Fillets in Breadcrumbs																									
Prawns																									
Salmon Steaks																									
Sardines																									
Scallops																									
Scampi in Breadcrumbs																									
Scottish Salmon Trout																									
Seafood Sticks																									
Shrimps																									
Smoked Cod Fillets																									

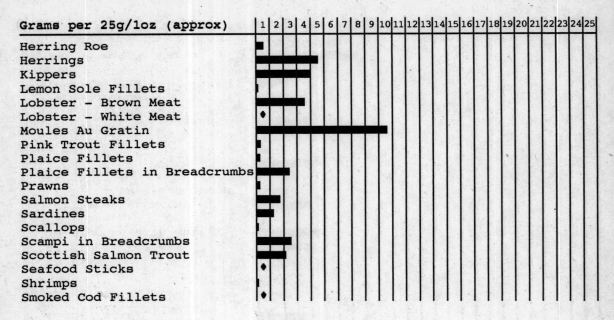

157

Smoked Haddock Fillets
Smoked Pacific Salmon
Smoked Scottish Salmon
Sprats
Squid
Swordfish
Trout
Whelks
Whiting

Frozen Fish
Cod Fillets
Cod Fillets – Skinless
Cod Portions
Coley Portions
Golden Haddock Cutlets
Haddock Fillets
Haddock Fillets – Skinless
Haddock Portion
Hake – Skinless
Kippered Mackerel

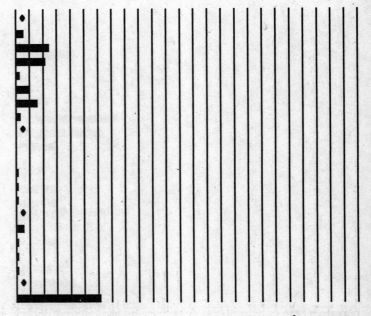

♦ = negligible

Grams per 25g/1oz (approx)

Item	1	2	3	4	5	6	7	8	9	10	11	12	13	14	15	16	17	18	19	20	21	22	23	24	25
Kippered Mackerel Fillets	███████																								
Lemon Sole Fillets	█																								
Plaice Fillets	█																								
Plaice Portions	█																								
Prawns	▏																								
Prawns for Cooking	▏																								
Rainbow Trout	██																								
Salmon Steaks	███																								
Salmon Tail Fillets	███																								
Smoked Cod Fillets	◆																								
Smoked Haddock Fillets	◆																								
Smoked Kipper Fillets	███																								
Smoked Mackerel	███████																								
Smoked Mackerel Fillets	████████																								
White Fish Fillets	█																								
White Fish Portions	█																								
Cod Fillets in Breadcrumbs	██																								
Cod Fillets in Ovencrisp Batter	█████																								

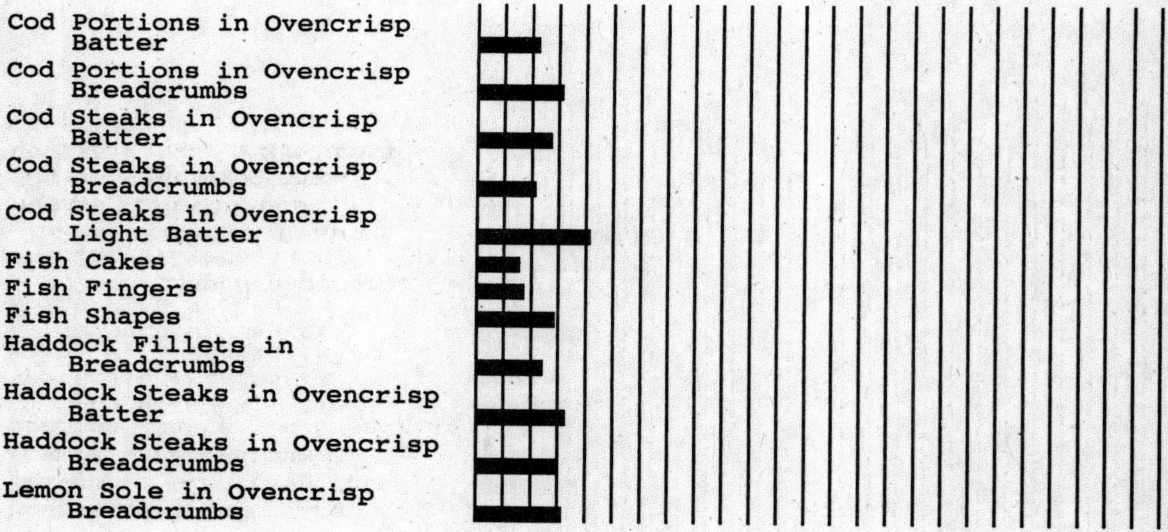

Cod Portions in Ovencrisp Batter	
Cod Portions in Ovencrisp Breadcrumbs	
Cod Steaks in Ovencrisp Batter	
Cod Steaks in Ovencrisp Breadcrumbs	
Cod Steaks in Ovencrisp Light Batter	
Fish Cakes	
Fish Fingers	
Fish Shapes	
Haddock Fillets in Breadcrumbs	
Haddock Steaks in Ovencrisp Batter	
Haddock Steaks in Ovencrisp Breadcrumbs	
Lemon Sole in Ovencrisp Breadcrumbs	

160

♦ = negligible

Grams per 25g/1oz (approx)	1	2	3	4	5	6	7	8	9	10	11	12	13	14	15	16	17	18	19	20	21	22	23	24	25
Ovencrisp Plaice with Prawn & Mushroom Filling	██████																								
Plaice Fillets in Breadcrumbs	█████																								
Plaice in Breadcrumbs	█████																								
Prawns in Ovencrisp Batter	███████																								
Scampi in Breadcrumbs	█████																								
Seafood Platter in Ovencrisp Breadcrumbs	████																								
White Fish Fingers	███																								
White Fish Steaks in Ovencrisp Batter	███████																								
White Fish Steaks in Ovencrisp Breadcrumbs	███████																								
Whiting Fillets in Breadcrumbs	█████																								
Cod in Butter Sauce	██																								
Cod in Parsley Sauce	█																								
Cod in Pastry with Cream Sauce	█████																								

161

Cod in Pastry with Prawn &
    Mushroom Sauce
Cod with Provencale Topping
Plaice Kiev

WAITROSE
Red Salmon
Pink Salmon
Sardines in Soya Oil
Sardines in Tomato Sauce
Sardines in Olive Oil
Sardines in Brine
Tuna in Oil
Whole Rainbow Trout
Whole Dover Sole
Trout with Stuffing
Trout with Mushroom & Onion
Cod Fillets
Haddock Fillets
Plaice Fillets
Lemon Sole Fillets

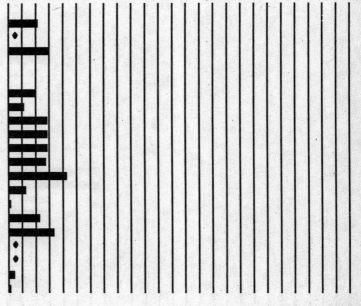

♦ = negligible

Grams per 25g/1oz (approx)	1	2	3	4	5	6	7	8	9	10	11	12	13	14	15	16	17	18	19	20	21	22	23	24	25
Trout Fillets																									
Salmon Steaks																									
Smoked Cod Fillets																									
Smoked Haddock Fillets																									
Whole Kippers																									
Cooked & Peeled Prawns																									
Whole Sliced Salmon																									
Smoked Salmon																									
Smoked Peppered Mackerel																									
Smoked Mackerel Fillets																									
Smoked Scotch Salmon																									
Breaded Cod Fillets																									
Breaded Haddock Fillets																									
Breaded Plaice Fillets																									
Coley Fillets																									
Golden Haddock Cutlets																									
Finnan Haddock																									
Boned Kippers																									
Chunky Cod Fillets																									

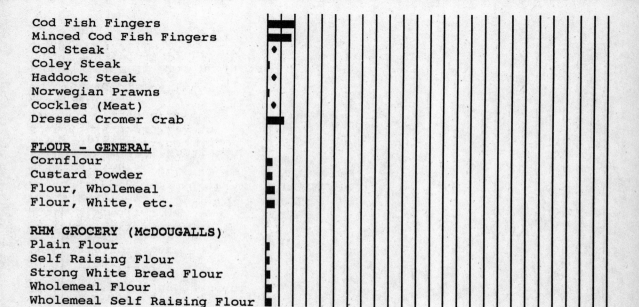

Cod Fish Fingers
Minced Cod Fish Fingers
Cod Steak
Coley Steak
Haddock Steak
Norwegian Prawns
Cockles (Meat)
Dressed Cromer Crab

FLOUR - GENERAL
Cornflour
Custard Powder
Flour, Wholemeal
Flour, White, etc.

RHM GROCERY (McDOUGALLS)
Plain Flour
Self Raising Flour
Strong White Bread Flour
Wholemeal Flour
Wholemeal Self Raising Flour

164

♦ = negligible

Grams per 25g/1oz (approx)	1	2	3	4	5	6	7	8	9	10	11	12	13	14	15	16	17	18	19	20	21	22	23	24	25

SAINSBURYS

100% Wholewheat Stoneground Flour	■																								
Plain Flour	■																								
Self Raising Flour	■																								
Strong Brown Flour	■																								

TESCO

Cornflour	♦																								
Plain	■																								
Self Raising	■																								
Stoneground 100% Wholewheat	■																								
Strong Plain	■																								
Strong Plain Brown	■																								

WAITROSE

Custard Powder	■																								
Super Fine Self Raising Flour	■																								
Super Fine Plain Flour	■																								

Strong White Plain Flour
Wholewheat Flour
Self Raising Flour
Wholemeal Breadcrumb
Natural Colour Breadcrumb

FROMAGE FRAIS - GENERAL
Creamy Fromage Frais
Fruit Fromage Frais
Low Fat Fromage Frais
Ordinary Fromage Frais

**NESTLE (Chambourcy Fromage
    Frais)**
Natural - Very Low Fat
Natural - Creamy
Fruit - Very Low Fat
Fruit - Creamy
Petit Fromage Frais with
    Fruit Puree

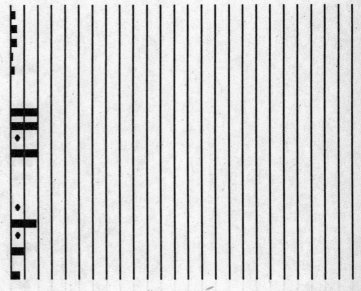

♦ = negligible

Grams per 25g/1oz (approx)	1	2	3	4	5	6	7	8	9	10	11	12	13	14	15	16	17	18	19	20	21	22	23	24	25
Mousse de Fromage Frais – Strawberry	██																								
Mamselle Sundae – Exotic Fruit	█																								
Hippotots Strawberry Dessert	███																								

SAINSBURYS

Fromage Frais with Fruit

	1	2	3	4	5	6	7	8	9	10	11	12	13	14	15	16	17	18	19	20	21	22	23	24	25
Apricot	██																								
Blackberry & Raspberry	██																								
Cherry	██																								
Peach & Strawberry	██																								
Raspberry	██																								
Strawberry	██																								
Virtually Fat Free Fromage Frais	◆																								
Low Fat Fromage Frais	██																								

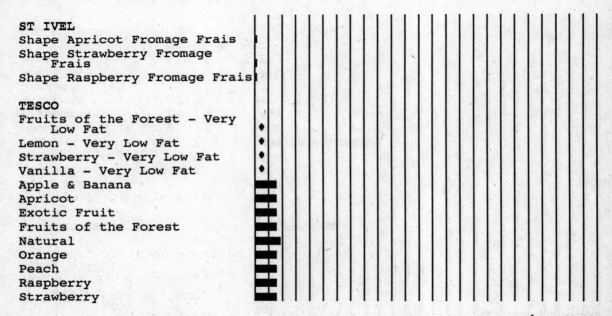

ST IVEL
Shape Apricot Fromage Frais
Shape Strawberry Fromage
    Frais
Shape Raspberry Fromage Frais

TESCO
Fruits of the Forest – Very
    Low Fat
Lemon – Very Low Fat
Strawberry – Very Low Fat
Vanilla – Very Low Fat
Apple & Banana
Apricot
Exotic Fruit
Fruits of the Forest
Natural
Orange
Peach
Raspberry
Strawberry

◆ = negligible

Grams per 25g/1oz (approx)	1	2	3	4	5	6	7	8	9	10	11	12	13	14	15	16	17	18	19	20	21	22	23	24	25
Strawberry & Vanilla	██																								
Natural – Very Low Fat	♦																								
FRUIT – GENERAL																									
Apples	♦																								
Apricots	♦																								
Avocado Pears	███████████																								
Bananas	♦																								
Bilberries	♦																								
Blackberries	♦																								
Cherries	♦																								
Cherries, Glacé	♦																								
Coconut – Flesh only	████████████																								
Coconut – Milk only	♦																								
Cranberries	♦																								
Currants	♦																								
Damsons	♦																								
Dates	♦																								
Figs	♦																								

```
Fruit Pie Filling
Fruit Salad
Gooseberries
Grapes
Grapefruit
Greengages
Guavas
Lemons
Loganberries
Lychees
Mandarin Oranges
Mangoes
Medlars
Melons
Mulberries
Nectarines
Olives
Oranges
Passion Fruit
Paw
Peaches
```

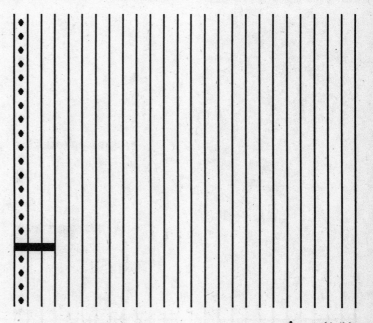

170

◆ = negligible

Grams per 25g/1oz (approx)	1	2	3	4	5	6	7	8	9	10	11	12	13	14	15	16	17	18	19	20	21	22	23	24	25
Pears	◆																								
Pineapple	◆																								
Plums	◆																								
Pomegranate	◆																								
Prunes	◆																								
Quinces	◆																								
Raisins	◆																								
Raspberries	◆																								
Rhubarb	◆																								
Strawberries	◆																								
Sultanas	◆																								
Tangerines	◆																								

CO-OP

Canned - in Juice
	1	2	3	4	5	6	7	8	9	10	11	12	13	14	15	16	17	18	19	20	21	22	23	24	25
Apricot Halves	◆																								
Fruit Cocktail	◆																								
Grapefruit Segments	◆																								

Mandarin Oranges ♦
Pear Halves ♦
Peach Slices ♦
Pineapple Slices/Chunks ♦
Prunes ♦
Raspberries ♦

Canned - Pie Fillings
Apple ♦
Apple & Blackberry ♦
Apple & Raspberry ♦
Blackcurrant ♦
Cherry ♦
Strawberry ♦
Strawberries ♦

Canned - in Syrup
Apricot Halves ♦
Fruit Cocktail ♦
Fruit Salad ♦
Grapefruit Segments ♦

♦ = negligible

Grams per 25g/1oz (approx)	1	2	3	4	5	6	7	8	9	10	11	12	13	14	15	16	17	18	19	20	21	22	23	24	25
Mandarins	◆																								
Pear Halves/Quarters	◆																								
Peach Slices/Halves	◆																								
Pineapple Slices/Chunks	◆																								
Plums Red/Golden	◆																								
Prunes	◆																								
Raspberries	◆																								
Rhubarb Pieces	◆																								
Strawberries	◆																								
Two Fruits	◆																								

SAINSBURYS

Fresh

	1	2	3	4	5	6	7	8	9	10	11	12	13	14	15	16	17	18	19	20	21	22	23	24	25
Apples - Cooking	◆																								
Apples Coxs	◆																								
Apples Golden Delicious	◆																								
Apples Granny Smith	◆																								
Apples Red Dessert	◆																								

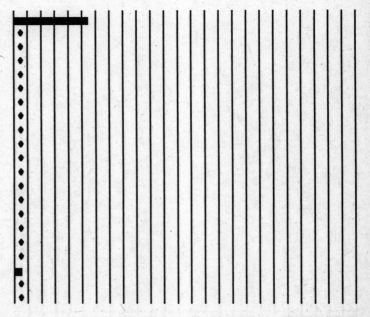

Avocado Pears
Bananas
Bilberries
Blackberries
Cherries
Cranberries
Damsons
Dates
Figs
Gooseberries
Grapefruit
Grapes – White
Grapes – Black
Greengages
Guavas
Kiwi Fruit
Kumquats
Lemons
Limes
Lychees
Mangoes

♦ = negligible

174

Grams per 25g/1oz (approx)	1	2	3	4	5	6	7	8	9	10	11	12	13	14	15	16	17	18	19	20	21	22	23	24	25
Melon Cantaloupe	◆																								
Melon Honeydew	◆																								
Melon Water	◆																								
Nectarines	◆																								
Oranges	◆																								
Passion Fruit	◆																								
Paw	◆																								
Pears Conference	◆																								
Pears Dessert	◆																								
Peaches	◆																								
Pineapple	◆																								
Plums – Dessert	◆																								
Rhubarb	◆																								
Strawberries	◆																								
Tangerines	◆																								
Canned – in Juice																									
Apricot Halves	◆																								
Grapefruit Segments	◆																								

Peach Slices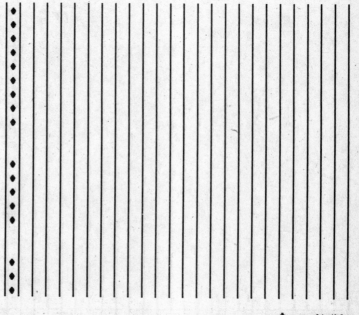
Pear Halves
Pear Quarters
Pineapple Pieces
Pineapple Slices
Prunes
Satsuma Oranges
Fruit Cocktail
Blackberries

Canned - Pie Filling
Apricot
Stewed Apple
Blackcurrant
Red Cherry
Swiss Black Cherry

Canned - in Syrup
Apricot Halves
Grapefruit Segments
Peach Halves/Slices

176

♦ = negligible

Grams per 25g/1oz (approx)	1	2	3	4	5	6	7	8	9	10	11	12	13	14	15	16	17	18	19	20	21	22	23	24	25
Pear Halves/Quarters	◆																								
Prunes	◆																								
Satsuma Oranges	◆																								
Fruit Cocktail	◆																								
Raspberries	◆																								
Strawberries	◆																								
Golden Plums	◆																								

TESCO

Fresh

	1	2	3	4	5	6	7	8	9	10	11	12	13	14	15	16	17	18	19	20	21	22	23	24	25
Apples - Bramley	◆																								
Apples - Cooking	◆																								
Apples - Coxs	◆																								
Apples - Golden Delicious	◆																								
Apples - Granny Smith	◆																								
Apples - Red Dessert	◆																								
Apples - Spartan	◆																								
Apples - Worcester	◆																								

Apricots
Bananas
Bilberries
Blackberries
Blackcurrants
Cantaloupe Melon
Cherries
Coconut, Flesh Only
Coconut, Milk Only
Cranberries
Damsons
Dessert Plums
Figs
Galia Melon
Gooseberries
Grapefruit
Grapes (Black)
Grapes (White)
Greengages
Lemons
Medlar

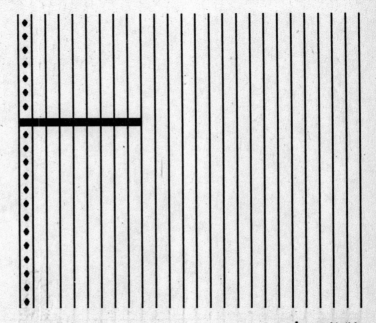

♦ = negligible

Grams per 25g/1oz (approx)	1	2	3	4	5	6	7	8	9	10	11	12	13	14	15	16	17	18	19	20	21	22	23	24	25
Nectarines	•																								
Ogen Melon	•																								
Oranges	•																								
Peaches	•																								
Pears	•																								
Pineapple	•																								
Redcurrants	•																								
Rhubarb, Stewed without Sugar	•																								
Rock Melon	•																								
Strawberries	•																								
Tangerines	•																								
Watermelon	•																								
Yellow Honeydew Melon	•																								
Exotic																									
Dates	•																								
Guava	•																								
Kiwi Fruit	•																								
Kumquat	•																								

```
Limes                   ■
Lychees                 ♦
Mango                   ♦
Ortanique               ♦
Passion Fruit           ♦
Paw (Papaya)            ♦
Pomegranate             ♦
Pomelo                  ♦
Ugli Fruit              ♦

Canned - in Juice
Fruit Cocktail          ♦
Grapefruit Segments     ♦
Peach Halves/Slices     ♦
Pear Halves/Slices      ♦
Pineapple Slices        ♦

Canned in Syrup
Fruit Cocktail          ♦
Golden Plums            ♦
Grapefruit Segments     ♦
```

♦ = negligible

Grams per 25g/1oz (approx)	1	2	3	4	5	6	7	8	9	10	11	12	13	14	15	16	17	18	19	20	21	22	23	24	25
Peach Halves/Slices	•																								
Pear Halves/Quarters	•																								
Pineapple Cubes/Fingers/Slices	•																								
Prunes	•																								
Raspberries	•																								
Strawberries	•																								
Canned – Pie Filling																									
Apple	•																								
Apple & Raspberry	•																								
Apple & Blackberry	•																								
Cherry	•																								
Gooseberry	•																								
Strawberry	•																								
Dried																									
Cake Fruit Mixture	•																								
Currants	•																								

Raisins	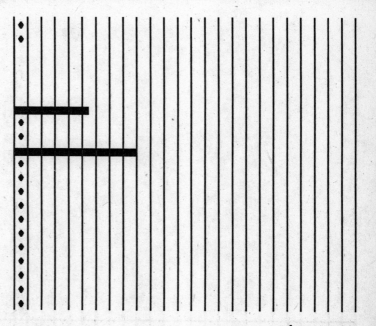
Sultanas	

WAITROSE

Fresh
Avocado Pears
Bananas
Cantaloupe Melons
Coconuts
Conference Pears
Fresh Figs
Grapefruit
Guava
Honeydew Melons
Lemons
Oranges
Passion Fruit
Paw
Pineapple
Plums

♦ = negligible

Grams per 25g/1oz (approx)	1	2	3	4	5	6	7	8	9	10	11	12	13	14	15	16	17	18	19	20	21	22	23	24	25
Raspberries	•																								
Rhubarb	•																								
Semi-Dried Figs	•																								
Semi-Dried Prunes	•																								
Semi-Dried Apricots	•																								
Strawberries	•																								

FRUIT JUICES & SOFT DRINKS - GENERAL

	1	2	3	4	5	6	7	8	9	10	11	12	13	14	15	16	17	18	19	20	21	22	23	24	25
Coca Cola	•																								
Grapefruit Juice	•																								
Lemonade	•																								
Lime Juice Cordial	•																								
Lucozade	•																								
Orange Drink	•																								
Orange Juice	•																								
Pineapple Juice	•																								
Ribena	•																								
Rosehip Syrup	•																								

Tomato Juice	◆
BOOTS	
High Juice - Lemon	◆
High Juice - Orange	◆
Lemon Barley Water	◆
Orange Barley Water	◆
Whole Lemon Drink	◆
Whole Orange Drink	◆
Instant Dried Skimmed Milk	▮
High Juice Tropical Fruit Squash	◆
Reduced Sugar Blackcurrant Drink	◆
Squeezed Orange Juice	◆
Freshly Pressed English Apple Juice	◆
Unsweetened Grapefruit Juice	◆
Unsweetened Pineapple Juice	◆
Pure English Apple Juice	◆

◆ = negligible

Grams per 25g/1oz (approx)	1	2	3	4	5	6	7	8	9	10	11	12	13	14	15	16	17	18	19	20	21	22	23	24	25
Apple & Blackcurrant Low Calorie Drink	•																								
Grapefruit Low Calorie Drink	•																								
Lemon Barley Low Calorie Drink	•																								
Less Sharp Low Calorie Lemon Juice	•																								
Shapers Apple & Blackcurrant	•																								
Shapers Citrus Fruit Drink	•																								
Shapers Cloudy Lemonade	•																								
NESTLE (Libbys)																									
Apple C Drink	•																								
Blackcurrant C Drink	•																								
Four Fruit C Drink	•																								
Grapefruit C Drink	•																								
Lemon & Lime C Drink	•																								
Moonshine Juice	•																								
Orange C Drink	•																								

Pineapple C Drink

Tomato Juice

Um Bongo Juice

SAINSBURYS

English Apple

Pure Jaffa Grapefruit

Traditional Lemon Crush

Pure Jaffa Orange

Pure Pineapple

Ruby Red Grapefruit

Mixers

American Ginger Ale

Bitter Lemon

Dry Ginger Ale

Low Calorie Tonic Water

Low Calorie Bitter Lemon

Low Calorie American Ginger
   Ale

Orange Spritzer

♦ = negligible

Grams per 25g/1oz (approx)	1	2	3	4	5	6	7	8	9	10	11	12	13	14	15	16	17	18	19	20	21	22	23	24	25
Ordinary Spritzer	•																								
Soda Water	•																								
Summer Fruit Spritzer	•																								
Tonic Water	•																								
Bottled Carbonates																									
Cream Soda	•																								
Cola	•																								
Diet Cola	•																								
Lemonade	•																								
Diet Lemonade	•																								
Dilutables																									
Blackcurrant Drink	•																								
High Juice Blackcurrant Squash	•																								
High Juice Lemon Squash	•																								
High Juice Lime Cordial	•																								
High Juice Orange Squash	•																								

Sugar Free Orange Drink ◆
Sugar Free Lemon Drink ◆

ST IVEL
Real Orange Juice ◆
Real Pineapple Juice ◆
Real Grapefruit Juice ◆
Real Apple Juice ◆
Exotic Juice ◆
Mediterranean Juice ◆
Premier Orange ◆
Premier Apple ◆
Mr Juicy – Orange ◆
Mr Juicy – Pineapple ◆
Mr Juicy – Grapefruit ◆
Mr Juicy – Apple ◆

TESCO
Cherryade ◆
Cola ◆
Cola (Can) ◆

◆ = negligible

Grams per 25g/1oz (approx)	1	2	3	4	5	6	7	8	9	10	11	12	13	14	15	16	17	18	19	20	21	22	23	24	25
Diet Cola	•																								
Diet Lemonade	•																								
Ginger Beer (Can)	•																								
Lemonade	•																								
Lemonade Shandy	•																								
Lemonade Shandy (Can)	•																								
Limeade	•																								
Orangeade	•																								
Traditional Lemonade	•																								
Carton																									
Apple & Blackcurrant	•																								
Blackcurrant	•																								
Mixed Fruit	•																								
Orange, Lemon & Pineapple	•																								
Whole Orange	•																								

Chilled
Caribbean Drink
Pacific Drink

Dilutables (concentrate)
Blackcurrant
Lemon & Lime
Lemon Barley
Lime Juice Cordial
Low Calorie Lemon
Low Calorie Orange
Orange
Orange & Peach
Orange, Lemon & Pineapple
Whole Lemon

Mixers
American Ginger Ale
Bitter Lemon
Dry Ginger Ale
Indian Tonic Water

♦ = negligible

Grams per 25g/1oz (approx)	1	2	3	4	5	6	7	8	9	10	11	12	13	14	15	16	17	18	19	20	21	22	23	24	25
Low Calorie Mixers	◆																								
Tonic Water	◆																								
Juices - Fresh																									
Apple	◆																								
Freshly Pressed Apple	◆																								
Grapefruit	◆																								
Orange	◆																								
Pineapple	◆																								
Juices - Longlife																									
Apple	◆																								
Grapefruit	◆																								
Orange	◆																								
Orange & Pineapple	◆																								
Pineapple	◆																								
Tomato	◆																								

WAITROSE
Blackcurrant Drink ♦
Cola ♦
Orange Squash (40% Juice) ♦
High Orange Squash ♦
Orange Drink ♦
Caribbean Drink ♦
Low Cal Drink ♦
Orange & Peach Drink ♦
Low Cal Lemon Drink ♦
Lemon Squash (40% Juice) ♦
Whole Lemon Drink ♦
Lemon Squash (60% Juice) ♦
Lemon Juice ♦
Lemon & Lime Drink ♦
Lemonade ♦
Sparkling Orange ♦
Old Fashioned Lemonade ♦
Baby Apple & Blackcurrant ♦
Baby Apple & Orange Juice ♦
Baby Rosehip Juice ♦

♦ = negligible

Grams per 25g/1oz (approx)	1	2	3	4	5	6	7	8	9	10	11	12	13	14	15	16	17	18	19	20	21	22	23	24	25

GAME – GENERAL

Grouse, Roast, weighed with bone	▪																								
Partridge:																									
Roast	▪▪																								
Roast, weighed with bone	▪																								
Pheasant:																									
Roast	▪▪▪																								
Roast, weighed with bone	▪▪																								
Pigeon:																									
Roast	▪▪▪▪																								
Roast, weighed with bone	▪																								
Hare:																									
Stewed	▪▪▪																								
Stewed, weighed with bone	▪▪																								
Rabbit:																									
Stewed	▪▪																								
Stewed weighed with bone	▪																								
Venison, Roast	▪▪																								

ICE CREAM – GENERAL
Choc Ice
Cornish Dairy
Vanilla Plain
Vanilla Soft Scoop

ICELAND
Chocolate Fudge Ripple Ice
 Cream
Vanilla Ice Cream
Neapolitan Ice Cream
Raspberry Ripple Ice Cream
White Vanilla Ice Cream
Black Cherry Ripple Ice Cream
Chocolate Ripple Ice Cream
Light Choc Ices
Dark Choc Ices
Double Choc Ices
Rum & Raisin Choc Ices
Assorted Ice Lollies
Vanilla Snow Ice Lollies

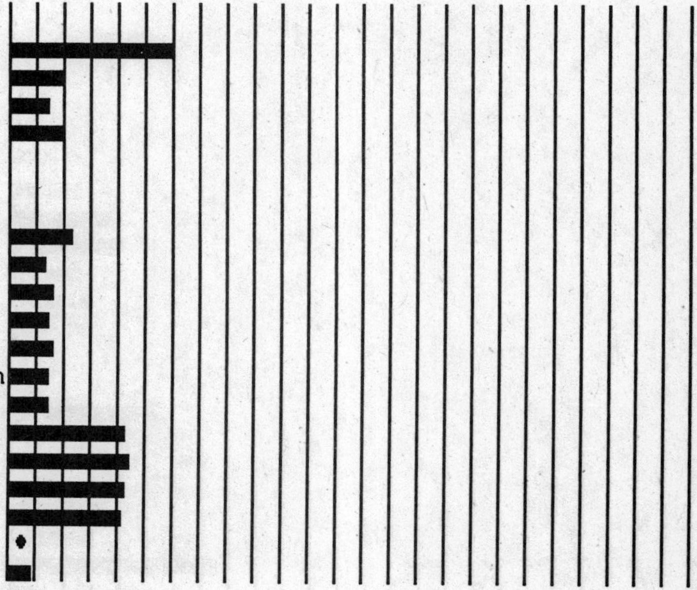

194

♦ = negligible

Grams per 25g/1oz (approx)

Scale: 1 2 3 4 5 6 7 8 9 10 11 12 13 14 15 16 17 18 19 20 21 22 23 24 25

Item	Approx. grams per 25g/1oz
Lemon & Lime Fruit Pops	~1
Choc Trebles	~8
Screwballs	~2
Dairy Ice Cream Cones	~3½
Dairy Ice Cream Cones with Choc & Nut	~4
Dairy Ice Cream Cones with Choc & Mint	~5
Strawberry Splits	~1½
Orange Ice Lollies	~½
Knickerbocker Glories	~2½
Strawberry Bombes	~3
Black Cherry Bombes	~3½
Devon Toffee Bombes	~4½
Double Choc Luxury Bombes	~4
Chocolate Orange Bombes	~3
Raspberry Bombes	~1
Black Forest Bombes	~1

195

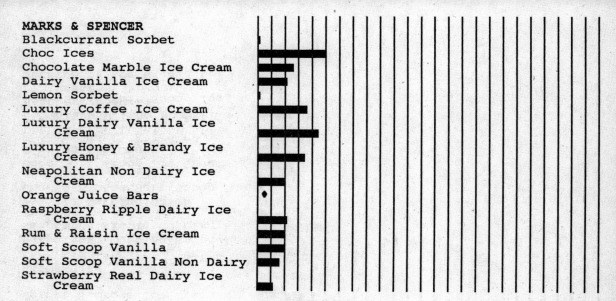

MARKS & SPENCER
Blackcurrant Sorbet
Choc Ices
Chocolate Marble Ice Cream
Dairy Vanilla Ice Cream
Lemon Sorbet
Luxury Coffee Ice Cream
Luxury Dairy Vanilla Ice Cream
Luxury Honey & Brandy Ice Cream
Neapolitan Non Dairy Ice Cream
Orange Juice Bars
Raspberry Ripple Dairy Ice Cream
Rum & Raisin Ice Cream
Soft Scoop Vanilla
Soft Scoop Vanilla Non Dairy
Strawberry Real Dairy Ice Cream

196

♦ = negligible

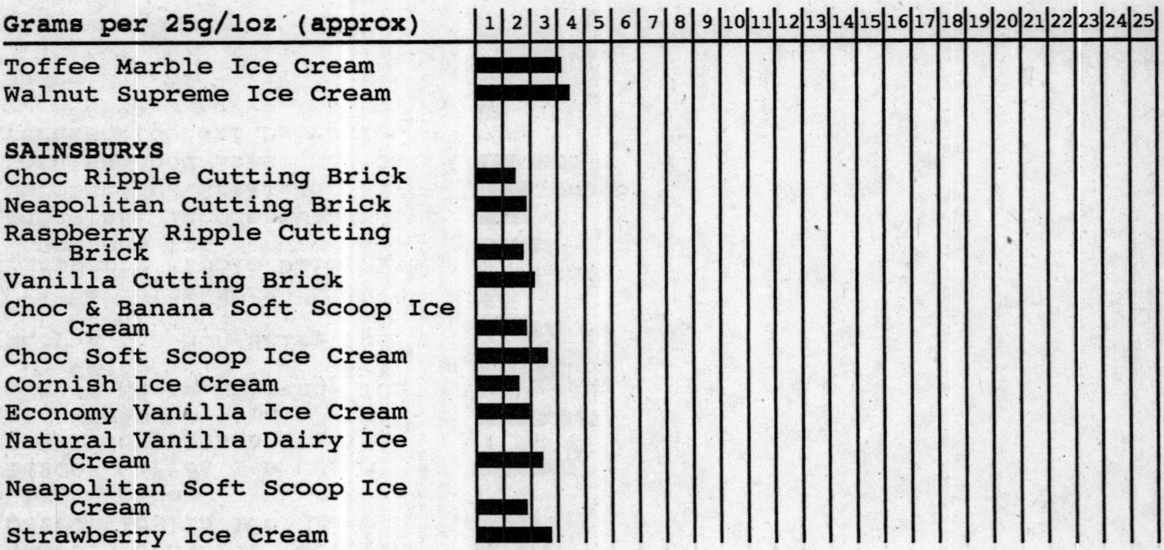

Grams per 25g/1oz (approx)	1	2	3	4	5	6	7	8	9	10	11	12	13	14	15	16	17	18	19	20	21	22	23	24	25

Toffee Marble Ice Cream ███
Walnut Supreme Ice Cream ████

SAINSBURYS
Choc Ripple Cutting Brick █▌
Neapolitan Cutting Brick ██
Raspberry Ripple Cutting Brick ██
Vanilla Cutting Brick ██▌
Choc & Banana Soft Scoop Ice Cream ██
Choc Soft Scoop Ice Cream ███
Cornish Ice Cream ██
Economy Vanilla Ice Cream █▌
Natural Vanilla Dairy Ice Cream ███
Neapolitan Soft Scoop Ice Cream ██
Strawberry Ice Cream ███

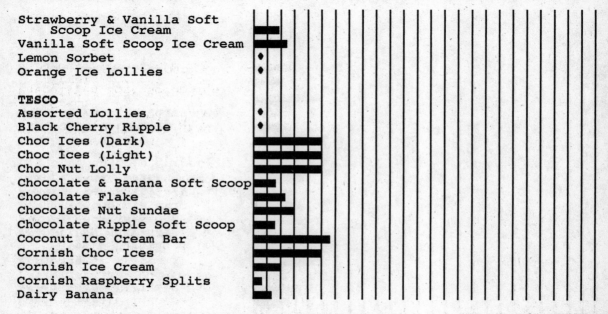

Strawberry & Vanilla Soft Scoop Ice Cream	
Vanilla Soft Scoop Ice Cream	
Lemon Sorbet	◆
Orange Ice Lollies	◆
TESCO	
Assorted Lollies	◆
Black Cherry Ripple	◆
Choc Ices (Dark)	
Choc Ices (Light)	
Choc Nut Lolly	
Chocolate & Banana Soft Scoop	
Chocolate Flake	
Chocolate Nut Sundae	
Chocolate Ripple Soft Scoop	
Coconut Ice Cream Bar	
Cornish Choc Ices	
Cornish Ice Cream	
Cornish Raspberry Splits	
Dairy Banana	

◆ = negligible

Grams per 25g/1oz (approx)

Food	Grams per 25g/1oz (approx)
Dairy Cornish	2.5
Dairy Strawberry	2
Dairy Vanilla	2.5
Fun Size Choc Ices	5
Ice Cream Roll	2
Knickerbocker Glory	1.5
Luxury Choc Ices	5
Luxury Chocolate Chip	3
Luxury French Style Vanilla	3
Luxury Maple Walnut	4
Mango & Mandarin Sorbet Whirls	2
Mint Choc Ices	5
Mint Chocolate Chip	2.5
Mint Neapolitan Soft Scoop	2
Muesli Ice Cream Bar	5
Neapolitan Brick	2.5
Neapolitan Soft Scoop	2
Orange Juice Lolly	0.5

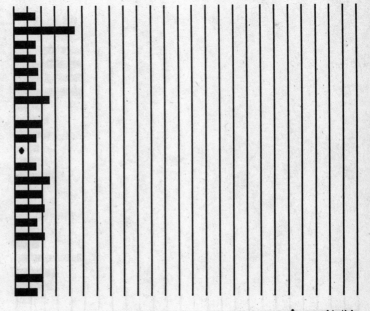

Peach Melba Soft Scoop
Peanut & Caramel Choc Bar
Raspberry Ripple
Raspberry Ripple Soft Scoop
Raspberry Sorbet Whirls
Strawberry & Cream Lollies
Strawberry & Vanilla Bombe
Strawberry & Vanilla Soft
    Scoop
Toffee Crunch
Tropical Fruit Juice Bar
Vanilla Brick
Vanilla Choc Flake
Vanilla Choc Nut
Vanilla Choc Nut Soft Scoop
Vanilla Pure White
Vanilla Soft Scoop

WAITROSE
American Vanilla Ice Cream
Black Cherry Ice Cream

200

♦ = negligible

Grams per 25g/1oz (approx)

Food	1	2	3	4	5	6	7	8	9	10	11	12	13	14	15	16	17	18	19	20	21	22	23	24	25
Blackcurrant Sorbet	◆																								
Choc Chip Ice Cream	███																								
Chocolate Ice Cream	███																								
Coffee Ice Cream	███																								
Cornish Dairy	██																								
Dairy Strawberry Ice Cream	██																								
Dairy Vanilla Ice Cream	██																								
Lemon Sorbet	◆																								
Neapolitan Ice Cream	███																								
Raspberry Ripple	███																								
Sliceable Vanilla	██																								
Soft Vanilla Ice Cream	██																								
Strawberry Ice Cream	███																								
Toffee/Almond Ice Cream	███																								
Vanilla Ice Cream	██																								
Milk Choc Ices	█████																								
Dark Choc Ices	█████																								
Mint Choc Ices	█████																								
Choc Chip Choc Ices	█████																								

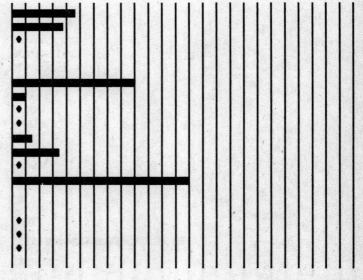

Neapolitan Choc Ices
Vanilla Choc Ice Lolly
Orange Ice Lolly

JAMS & PRESERVES - GENERAL
Chocolate Spread
Honeycomb
Honey in jars
Jam
Lemon Curd, Starch Based
Lemon Curd, Home Made
Marmalade
Peanut Butter

BOOTS
Honey - Acacia Blossom
Honey - Pure Clear
Honey - Pure Set

♦ = negligible

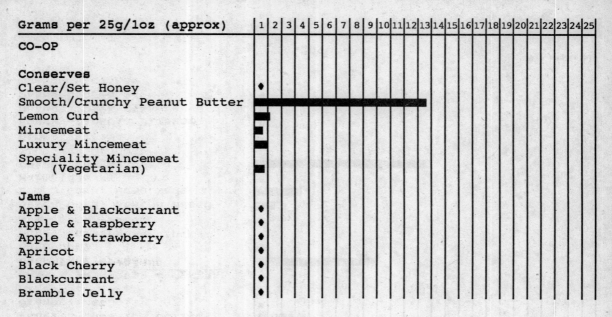

Grams per 25g/1oz (approx)	1	2	3	4	5	6	7	8	9	10	11	12	13	14	15	16	17	18	19	20	21	22	23	24	25
CO-OP																									
Conserves																									
Clear/Set Honey	♦																								
Smooth/Crunchy Peanut Butter	█	█	█	█	█	█	█	█	█	█	█	█	█												
Lemon Curd	█																								
Mincemeat	█																								
Luxury Mincemeat	█																								
Speciality Mincemeat (Vegetarian)	█																								
Jams																									
Apple & Blackcurrant	♦																								
Apple & Raspberry	♦																								
Apple & Strawberry	♦																								
Apricot	♦																								
Black Cherry	♦																								
Blackcurrant	♦																								
Bramble Jelly	♦																								

203

Damson

Ginger & Orange

Mixed Fruit

Pineapple

Plum

Raspberry Seedless

Raspberry

Strawberry Whole Fruit

Strawberry Puree

Strawberry

Marmalade

Coarse Cut Orange

Fine Cut Orange

Fine Cut Lemon

Fine Cut Lime

Mature Thick Cut Orange

Orange Shred

Orange Seedless

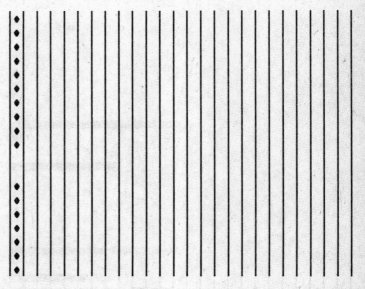

♦ = negligible

Grams per 25g/1oz (approx)	1	2	3	4	5	6	7	8	9	10	11	12	13	14	15	16	17	18	19	20	21	22	23	24	25
SAINSBURYS																									
Smooth Peanut Butter	████████████																								
Chocolate Hazelnut Spread	███████▊																								
Chocolate Spread	▌																								
Lemon Curd	█																								
TESCO																									
Conserves - all flavours	◆																								
Ginger Preserve	◆																								
Golden Syrup	◆																								
Hazelnut Chocolate Spread	████████																								
Honey	◆																								
Lemon Curd	█																								
Smooth/Crunchy Peanut Butter	█████████████																								
Jam																									
Apricot	◆																								
Blackcherry	◆																								
Blackcurrant	◆																								

Bramble Jelly
Damson
Pineapple
Plum
Raspberry
Strawberry

Marmalade
Fine Cut Orange
Lemon Shred
Lime Shred
Mature Thick Cut Orange
Orange Shred
Thick Cut Orange

WAITROSE

Conserves
Hazelnut Chocolate Spread
Lemon Curd
Lemon Cheese

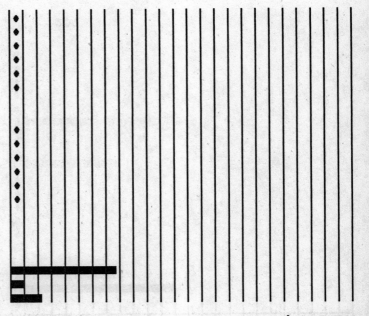

♦ = negligible

Grams per 25g/1oz (approx)	1	2	3	4	5	6	7	8	9	10	11	12	13	14	15	16	17	18	19	20	21	22	23	24	25
Molasses	●																								
Smooth/Crunchy Peanut Butter	██	██	██	██	██	██	██	██	██	██	██	██	██												
Savoury Spread	●																								
Fruit Spreads																									
Apricot	●																								
Bitter Orange	●																								
Blackcurrant	●																								
Raspberry	●																								
Strawberry	●																								
Honey																									
Acacia Honey	●																								
Australian Honey	●																								
Australian Clear Honey	●																								
Canadian Honey	●																								
Clear/Set Honey	●																								
English Honey	●																								
Greek Honey	●																								

Mexican Set Honey
Tasmanian Honey

Jam
Apricot
Black Cherry
Blackcurrant
Bramble Jelly
Ginger
Morello Cherry
Pineapple
Raspberry
Reduced Sugar Blackcurrant
Reduced Sugar Apricot
Reduced Sugar Raspberry
Seedless Raspberry
Strawberry
Victoria Plum

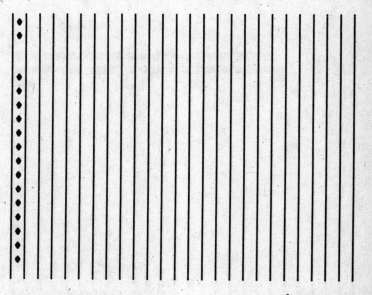

◆ = negligible

Grams per 25g/1oz (approx)	1	2	3	4	5	6	7	8	9	10	11	12	13	14	15	16	17	18	19	20	21	22	23	24	25

Marmalade
Fresh Grapefruit
Fresh Orange
Lemon & Lime Shred
Lemon Shred
Lime Shred
Orange Thin Cut
Orange Shred
Reduced Sugar Thin Cut Orange
Thick Cut 3 Fruits
Thick Cut

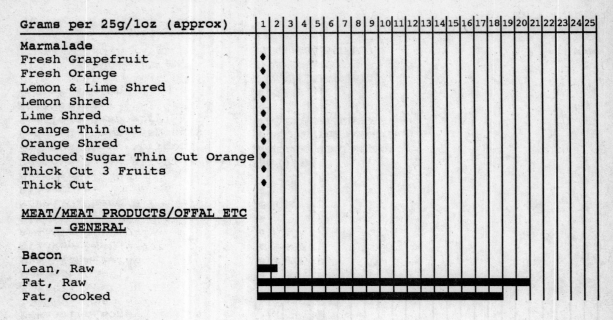

<u>**MEAT/MEAT PRODUCTS/OFFAL ETC**</u>
     <u>**- GENERAL**</u>

Bacon
Lean, Raw
Fat, Raw
Fat, Cooked

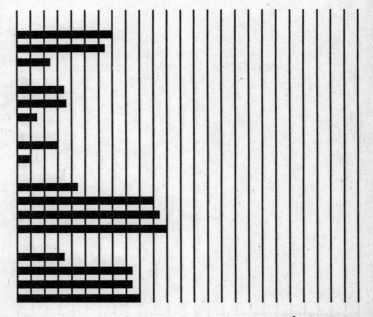

Collar Joint:
Raw, Lean & Fat
Boiled, Lean & Fat
Boiled, Lean only
Gammon Joint:
Raw, Lean & Fat
Boiled, Lean & Fat
Boiled, Lean only
Gammon Rashers:
Grilled, Lean & Fat
Grilled, Lean only
Rashers, Fried:
Lean only
Back, Lean & Fat
Middle, Lean & Fat
Streaky, Lean & Fat
Rashers, Grilled:
Lean only
Back, Lean & Fat
Middle, Lean & Fat
Streaky, Lean & Fat

♦ = negligible

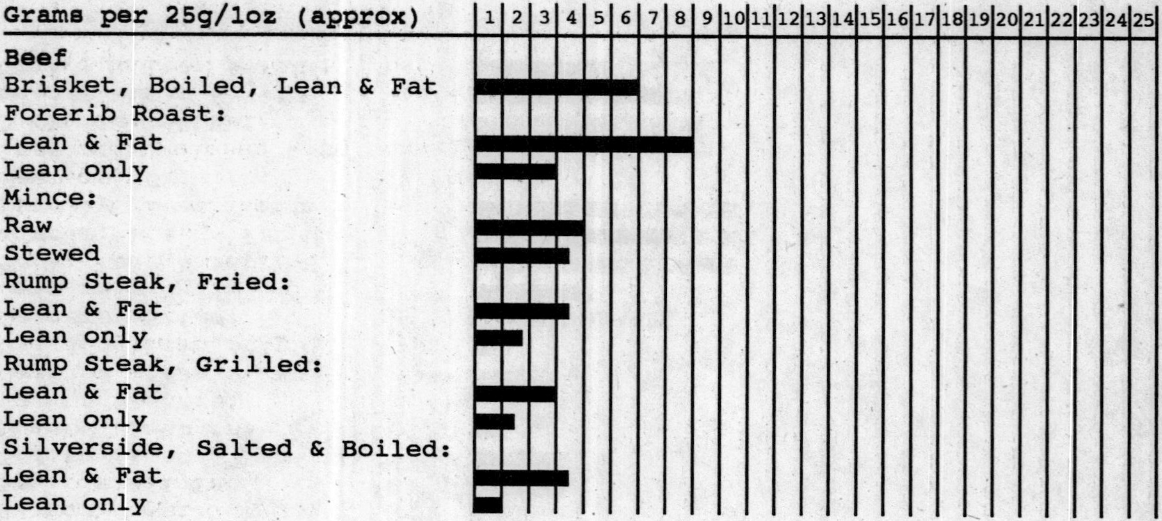
Grams per 25g/1oz (approx)
1 2 3 4 5 6 7 8 9 10 11 12 13 14 15 16 17 18 19 20 21 22 23 24 25
Beef
Brisket, Boiled, Lean & Fat
Forerib Roast:
Lean & Fat
Lean only
Mince:
Raw
Stewed
Rump Steak, Fried:
Lean & Fat
Lean only
Rump Steak, Grilled:
Lean & Fat
Lean only
Silverside, Salted & Boiled:
Lean & Fat
Lean only

Sirloin, Roast or Grilled:
Lean & Fat
Lean only
Stewing Steak:
Stewed, Lean & Fat
Topside Roast:
Lean & Fat
Lean only

Lamb
Breast, Roast:
Lean & Fat
Lean only
Chops, Loin, Grilled:
Lean & Fat
Lean & Fat weighed with bone
Lean only
Lean only weighed with bone
Cutlets, Grilled:
Lean & Fat
Lean & Fat weighed with bone

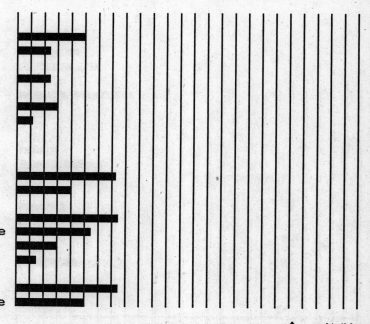

212

♦ = negligible

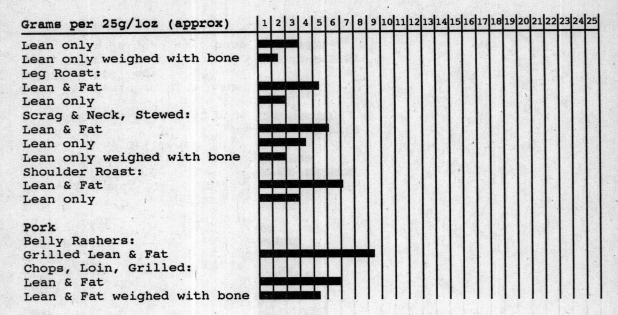

Lean only
Lean only weighed with fat &
     bone
Leg Roast:
Lean & Fat
Lean only

Veal
Cutlet, Fried
Fillet, Roast

Canned Meat
Corned Beef
Ham
Ham & Pork, Chopped
Luncheon Meat
Stewed Steak with Gravy
Tongue
Veal, Jellied

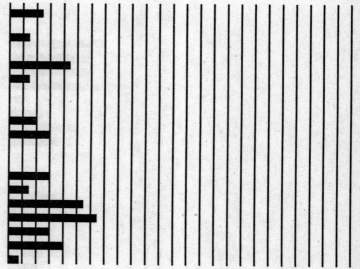

♦ = negligible

Grams per 25g/1oz (approx)	1	2	3	4	5	6	7	8	9	10	11	12	13	14	15	16	17	18	19	20	21	22	23	24	25

Cooked Meat

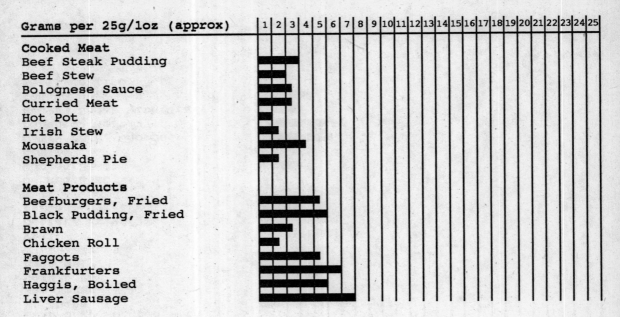

Beef Steak Pudding
Beef Stew
Bolognese Sauce
Curried Meat
Hot Pot
Irish Stew
Moussaka
Shepherds Pie

Meat Products
Beefburgers, Fried
Black Pudding, Fried
Brawn
Chicken Roll
Faggots
Frankfurters
Haggis, Boiled
Liver Sausage

Meat Paste
Polony
Salami
Sausages – Beef:
Fried
Grilled
Sausages – Pork:
Fried
Grilled
Saveloy
White Pudding

Offal
Brain:
Calf, Boiled
Lamb, Boiled
Heart:
Sheep, Roast
Ox, Stewed

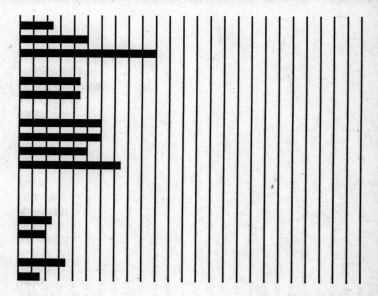

216

♦ = negligible

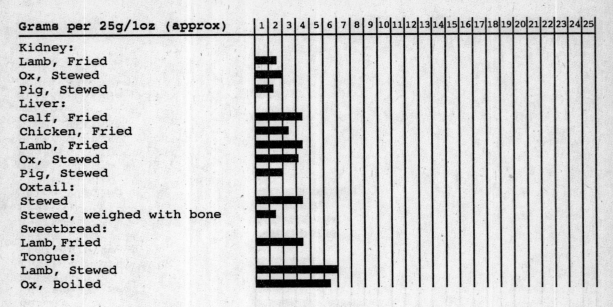

Grams per 25g/1oz (approx)	1	2	3	4	5	6	7	8	9	10	11	12	13	14	15	16	17	18	19	20	21	22	23	24	25

Kidney:
Lamb, Fried
Ox, Stewed
Pig, Stewed
Liver:
Calf, Fried
Chicken, Fried
Lamb, Fried
Ox, Stewed
Pig, Stewed
Oxtail:
Stewed
Stewed, weighed with bone
Sweetbread:
Lamb, Fried
Tongue:
Lamb, Stewed
Ox, Boiled

Tripe:
Stewed

CAMPBELLS
Beef Stew
Steak & Kidney Stew
Chicken Stew
Irish Stew
Meatballs with Beans
Meatballs with Pasta
Meatballs in Barbecue Sauce
Meatballs in Tomato Sauce
Meatballs in Gravy
Meatballs in Onion Gravy
Chicken Curry
Beef Curry
Chilli Con Carne
Chicken & Pasta Casserole
Vegetable Casserole
Minced Beef & Vegetables

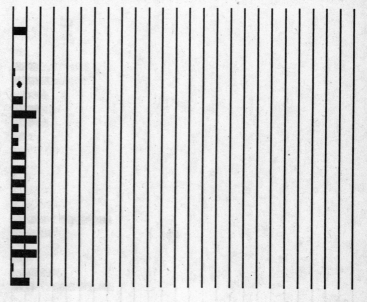

218

♦ = negligible

Grams per 25g/1oz (approx)	1	2	3	4	5	6	7	8	9	10	11	12	13	14	15	16	17	18	19	20	21	22	23	24	25
CO-OP																									
Chopped Ham with Pork								8																	
Hot Dog Sausages				3.5																					
Irish Stew	1																								
Minced Beef with Onions in Gravy			3																						
Pork Luncheon Meat								8																	
Steak Chunks in Rich Gravy	1																								
ICELAND																									
Beef																									
Beef Loaf	1.5																								
Braising Steak		2.5																							
Diced Steak & Kidney		2																							
Diced Steak		2.5																							
Diced Beef Steak		2.5																							
Diced Lean & Tender Steak		2																							
15 Minute Mince		2																							

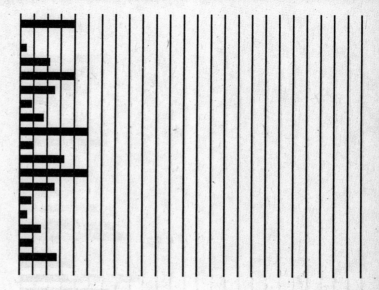

Economy Mince	
Extra Lean & Tender Minced Steak	
Free Flow Mince Steak	
Free Flow Mince	
Lean Braising Steak	
Peppered Steaks	
Premium Diced Steak	
Ready Carved Beef Joint	
Seasoned Steaks	
Silverside	
Slowcook Roasting Joint	
Stewing Steak	
Super Value Minced Beef	
Super Value Beef & Kidney	
Tenderised Sirloin Steaks	
Tenderised Rump Steaks	
Topside Rump	

220

◆ = negligible

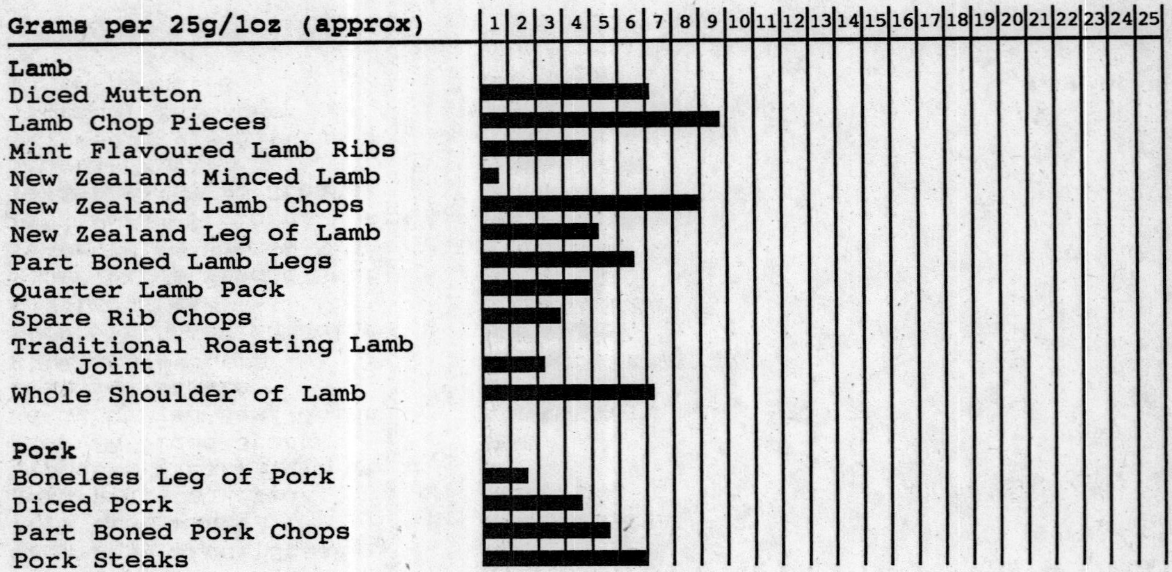

Grams per 25g/1oz (approx)

	1	2	3	4	5	6	7	8	9	10	11	12	13	14	15	16	17	18	19	20	21	22	23	24	25

Lamb
Diced Mutton ▇▇▇▇▇▇ (≈6)
Lamb Chop Pieces ▇▇▇▇▇▇▇▇▇ (≈9)
Mint Flavoured Lamb Ribs ▇▇▇▇ (≈4)
New Zealand Minced Lamb ▇ (≈1)
New Zealand Lamb Chops ▇▇▇▇▇▇▇▇ (≈8)
New Zealand Leg of Lamb ▇▇▇▇▇ (≈5)
Part Boned Lamb Legs ▇▇▇▇▇▇ (≈6)
Quarter Lamb Pack ▇▇▇▇ (≈4)
Spare Rib Chops ▇▇▇ (≈3)
Traditional Roasting Lamb
    Joint ▇▇ (≈2)
Whole Shoulder of Lamb ▇▇▇▇▇▇▇ (≈7)

Pork
Boneless Leg of Pork ▇▇ (≈2)
Diced Pork ▇▇▇▇ (≈4)
Part Boned Pork Chops ▇▇▇▇▇ (≈5)
Pork Steaks ▇▇▇▇▇▇ (≈6)

Pork Savoury Roast
Pork Loin Chops
Pork Chops
Pork Kebabs with Peppers
Pork Chop Pieces
Pork Belly Slices
Traditional Roasting Pork
    Joint

Meat Products
100% Beefburgers
Bacon Burgers
Bacon Burgers with Cheese
Bacon & Egg Burgers
Barbecue Relish Burgers
Beef Burgers
Burger Fingers
Cheeseburgers
Chinese Style Ribsteaks
Cocktail Sausages
Diced Rabbit

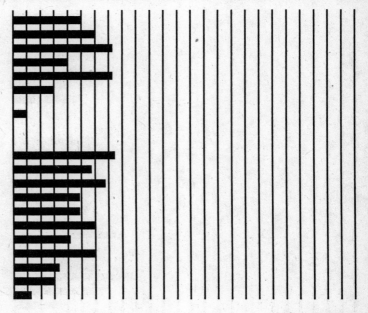

♦ = negligible

Grams per 25g/1oz (approx)

Food	Grams per 25g/1oz (approx)
Faggots in Rich Gravy	~4
Faggots in Cider Sauce with Apple	~3.5
Grillsteaks	~7
Liver & Onions	~1
Low Fat Beefburgers	~4.5
Pork Sausage Meat	~6
Quarter Pounders	~5.5
Quick Cook Beef Cubes	~5
Ribsteaks	~5
Thick Pork & Herb Sausage	~3.5
Tikka Ribsteaks	~5
Ready Meals	
Beef Stew & Dumplings	~1
Beef Sandwichsteaks	~6.5
Beef Curry with Rice	~2
Chilli Con Carne with Rice	~2
Chinese Pork Chop Suey	~4.5

Chinese Beef in Oyster Sauce

Chinese Beef in Black Bean
    Sauce

Chinese Sweet & Sour Pork

Indian Lamb Rogan Josh

Indian Beef Madras

Lancashire Hotpot

Minced Beef with Vegetable
    in Gravy

Minced Beef & Vegetable
    Hotpot

Sliced Beef in Gravy

Steak in Red Wine Sauce

MARKS & SPENCER

Beef
Braising Steak
Flash Fry Steak
Forerib Joint/Rib Eye Steak
Ground Beef

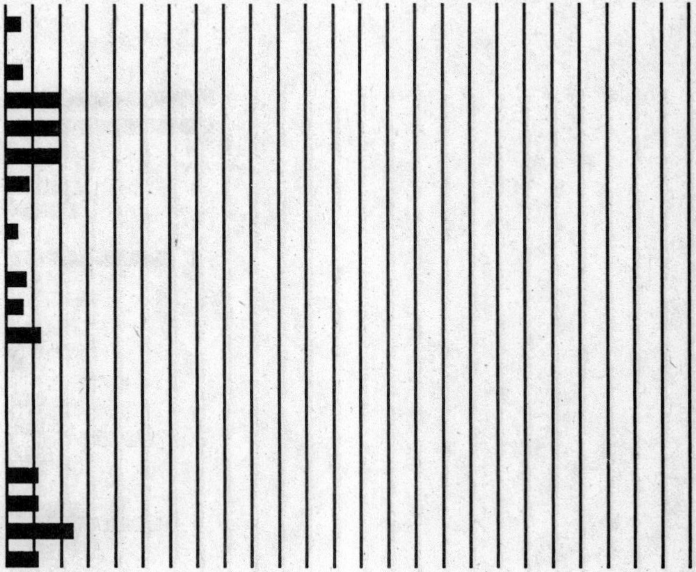

◆ = negligible

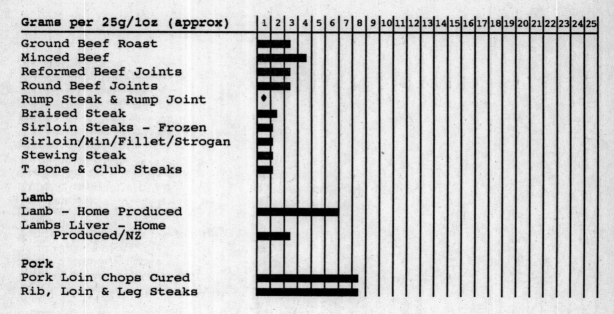

Grams per 25g/1oz (approx)	1	2	3	4	5	6	7	8	9	10	11	12	13	14	15	16	17	18	19	20	21	22	23	24	25
Ground Beef Roast																									
Minced Beef																									
Reformed Beef Joints																									
Round Beef Joints																									
Rump Steak & Rump Joint																									
Braised Steak																									
Sirloin Steaks - Frozen																									
Sirloin/Min/Fillet/Strogan																									
Stewing Steak																									
T Bone & Club Steaks																									

Lamb

Lamb - Home Produced																									
Lambs Liver - Home Produced/NZ																									

Pork

Pork Loin Chops Cured																									
Rib, Loin & Leg Steaks																									

225

Cooked Meats

Corned Beef
Bavarian Ham
Danish Ham
Half Ham on the Bone
Ham - Dry Cured Italian
Ham Joints - Bavarian
Honey Roast Ham - Thin Sliced
Roasted Ham Slices
Roasted Ham Joints
Cured Pork Roast with Herbs
Cured Pork - Chopped
Cured Salt Beef
Cured Pork Shoulder
Pork Tongue with Gelatine
Pork Loin - Roast & Sliced
Pork Tongue - Pressed & Sliced
Pork-Chopped Cured Thin Sliced

◆ = negligible

226

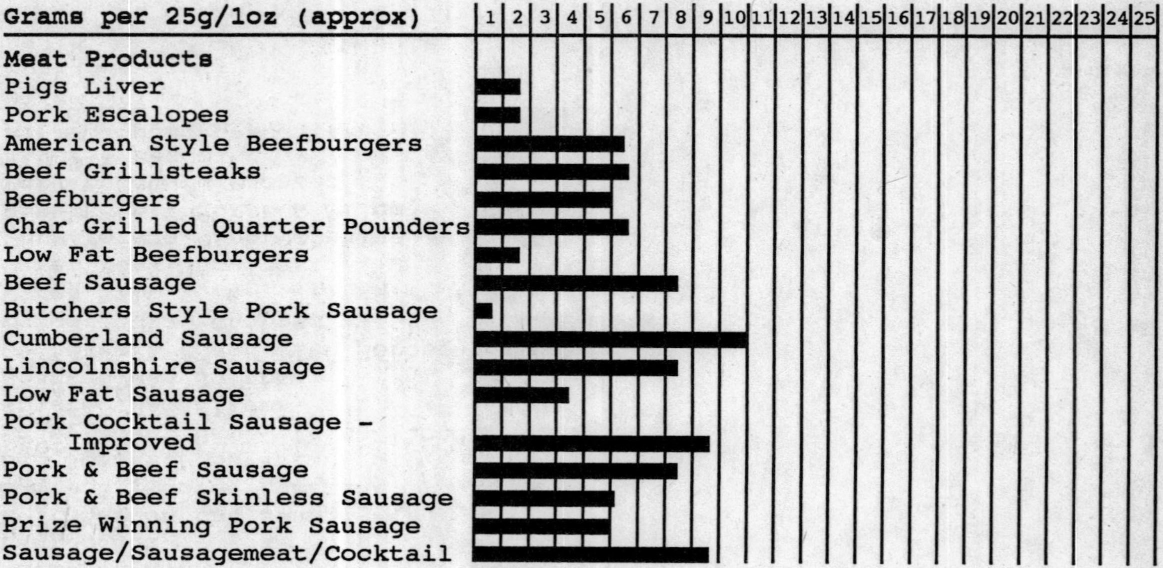

Grams per 25g/1oz (approx)

Meat Products

Product	Grams per 25g/1oz (approx)
Pigs Liver	2
Pork Escalopes	2
American Style Beefburgers	6
Beef Grillsteaks	7
Beefburgers	6
Char Grilled Quarter Pounders	6
Low Fat Beefburgers	3
Beef Sausage	8
Butchers Style Pork Sausage	1
Cumberland Sausage	10
Lincolnshire Sausage	8
Low Fat Sausage	4
Pork Cocktail Sausage – Improved	9
Pork & Beef Sausage	8
Pork & Beef Skinless Sausage	7
Prize Winning Pork Sausage	6
Sausage/Sausagemeat/Cocktail	9

227

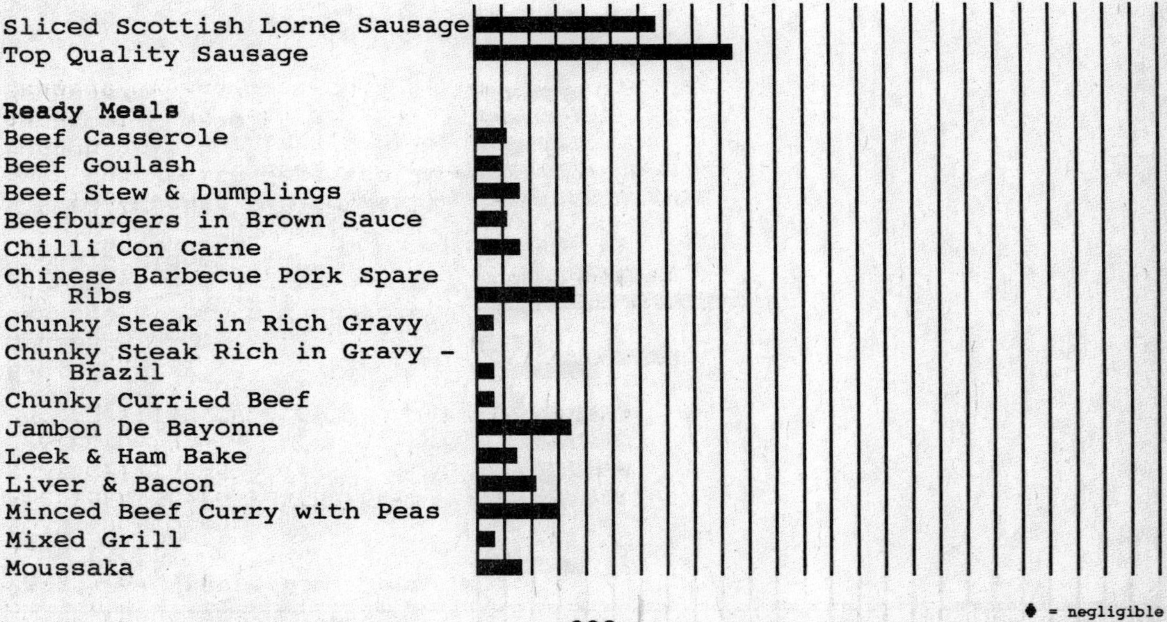

Sliced Scottish Lorne Sausage

Top Quality Sausage

Ready Meals

Beef Casserole

Beef Goulash

Beef Stew & Dumplings

Beefburgers in Brown Sauce

Chilli Con Carne

Chinese Barbecue Pork Spare
   Ribs

Chunky Steak in Rich Gravy

Chunky Steak Rich in Gravy –
   Brazil

Chunky Curried Beef

Jambon De Bayonne

Leek & Ham Bake

Liver & Bacon

Minced Beef Curry with Peas

Mixed Grill

Moussaka

228

◆ = negligible

Grams per 25g/1oz (approx)	1	2	3	4	5	6	7	8	9	10	11	12	13	14	15	16	17	18	19	20	21	22	23	24	25
Pancake – Cheese/Ham, Beer Batter	▓	▓	▓	▓																					
Roti De Boeuf	◆																								
Spring Roll – Chinese Style	▓	▓																							
Steak & Kidney Pie Meal	▓	▓	▓																							
NESTLE (Cook in Pot)																									
Lamb Ragout	▓	▓																								
Madras Curry	▓	▓	▓	▓																					
Moussaka	▓	▓	▓																							
Sausage & Tomato Casserole	▓	▓																								
Shepherds Pie	◆																									
Steak & Kidney	▓	▓	▓																							
NESTLE (Crosse & Blackwell)																									
Beef Curry with Separate Rice	▓																									
London Grill	▓	▓																								
Macaroni Cheese	▓	▓	▓																							
Moussaka	▓	▓	▓	▓																					

229

Prawn Curry
Roast Beef in Gravy
Tagliatelle in Cream &
      Cheese Sauce
Toad-in-the-Hole
Ham & Beef Roll
Ham & Chicken Roll
Ham & Tongue Roll
Ham & Turkey Roll

NESTLE (Findus)
Beef Madras Curry
Beef Oriental
Beef Stroganoff
Beef Teriyaki
Cannelloni
Cumberland Pie
Lasagne
Real Beefburgers
All Beef Quarterpounders
Beef Grill Steaks

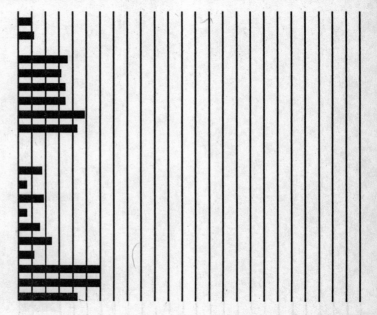

♦ = negligible

Grams per 25g/1oz (approx)	1	2	3	4	5	6	7	8	9	10	11	12	13	14	15	16	17	18	19	20	21	22	23	24	25
Lean Beefburgers	███																								
Lean Beef Grillados	███																								
Chilli Beef Grillados	█████																								
NESTLE (Findus Lean Cuisine)																									
Beef & Pork Cannelloni	▌																								
Beef Italienne	▌																								
Beef Julienne	▎																								
Beef Provencale	█																								
Beef Satay	▌																								
OXO Slim-A-Meal																									
Beef Risotto	▌																								
Chow Mein	▌																								
Paella	▌																								
SAINSBURYS																									

Bacon

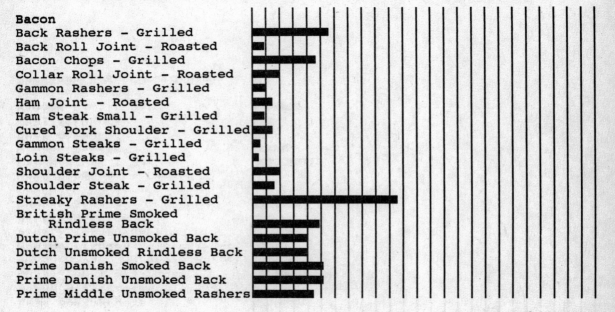

Back Rashers - Grilled
Back Roll Joint - Roasted
Bacon Chops - Grilled
Collar Roll Joint - Roasted
Gammon Rashers - Grilled
Ham Joint - Roasted
Ham Steak Small - Grilled
Cured Pork Shoulder - Grilled
Gammon Steaks - Grilled
Loin Steaks - Grilled
Shoulder Joint - Roasted
Shoulder Steak - Grilled
Streaky Rashers - Grilled
British Prime Smoked
    Rindless Back
Dutch Prime Unsmoked Back
Dutch Unsmoked Rindless Back
Prime Danish Smoked Back
Prime Danish Unsmoked Back
Prime Middle Unsmoked Rashers

◆ = negligible

232

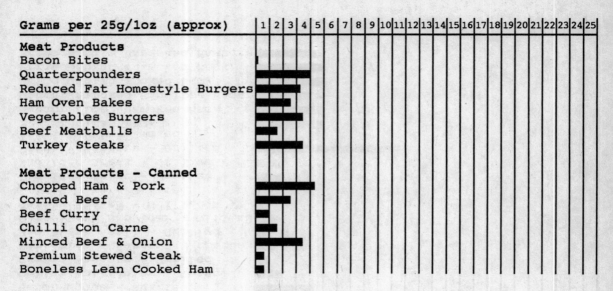

Grams per 25g/1oz (approx)	1	2	3	4	5	6	7	8	9	10	11	12	13	14	15	16	17	18	19	20	21	22	23	24	25
Meat Products																									
Bacon Bites																									
Quarterpounders																									
Reduced Fat Homestyle Burgers																									
Ham Oven Bakes																									
Vegetables Burgers																									
Beef Meatballs																									
Turkey Steaks																									
Meat Products – Canned																									
Chopped Ham & Pork																									
Corned Beef																									
Beef Curry																									
Chilli Con Carne																									
Minced Beef & Onion																									
Premium Stewed Steak																									
Boneless Lean Cooked Ham																									

233

Ready Meals - Chilled
Barbecue Spare Ribs
Beef & Veg Stew with
    Dumplings
Gobi Aloo Sag
Traditional Beef Hot Pot
Pineapple Chicken & Barbecue
    Beef
Minced Beef Cobbler
Roast Beef in Gravy

TESCO

Bacon
Prime Bacon Joint
Bacon Joint/Steaks
Gammon Joint
Gammon Steak
Collar Joint
Hock Joint
Knuckle

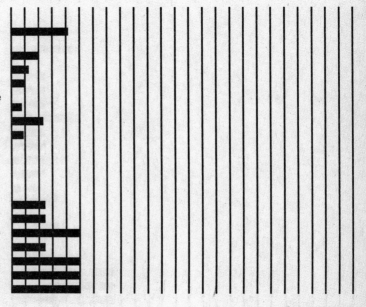

♦ = negligible

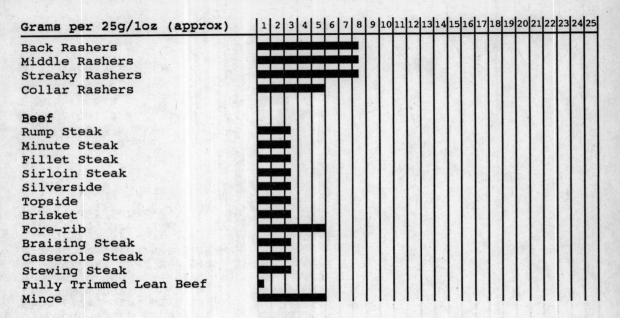

Grams per 25g/1oz (approx)	1	2	3	4	5	6	7	8	9	10	11	12	13	14	15	16	17	18	19	20	21	22	23	24	25
Back Rashers																									
Middle Rashers																									
Streaky Rashers																									
Collar Rashers																									
Beef																									
Rump Steak																									
Minute Steak																									
Fillet Steak																									
Sirloin Steak																									
Silverside																									
Topside																									
Brisket																									
Fore-rib																									
Braising Steak																									
Casserole Steak																									
Stewing Steak																									
Fully Trimmed Lean Beef																									
Mince																									

235

Lean Mince

Lamb
Leg
Shoulder
Scrag/Neck
Breast
Lamb Chops
Chump Chops
Mince
Fully Trimmed Lean Lamb

Offal
Heart
Kidney
Liver
Oxtail

Pork
Fillet/Tenderloin
Shoulder

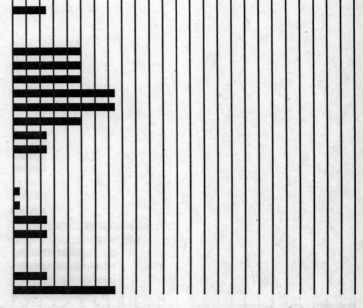

♦ = negligible

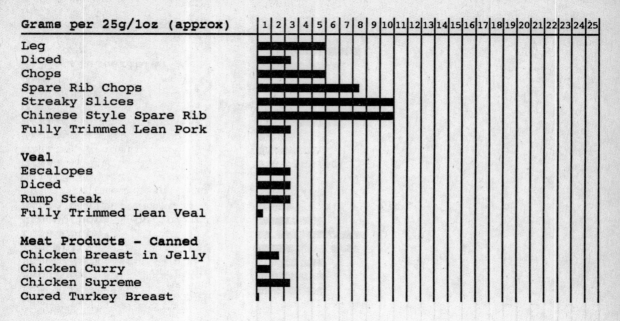

Grams per 25g/1oz (approx)

Cut	1 2 3 4 5 6 7 8 9 10 11 12 13 14 15 16 17 18 19 20 21 22 23 24 25
Leg	▇▇▇▇▇
Diced	▇▇▇
Chops	▇▇▇▇▇
Spare Rib Chops	▇▇▇▇▇▇▇▇
Streaky Slices	▇▇▇▇▇▇▇▇▇▇▇
Chinese Style Spare Rib	▇▇▇▇▇▇▇▇▇▇
Fully Trimmed Lean Pork	▇▇▇
Veal	
Escalopes	▇▇▇
Diced	▇▇▇
Rump Steak	▇▇▇
Fully Trimmed Lean Veal	▏
Meat Products – Canned	
Chicken Breast in Jelly	▇▇
Chicken Curry	▇▇
Chicken Supreme	▇▇▇
Cured Turkey Breast	▏

Economy Chicken & Vegetable
     Curry
Economy Irish Stew
Economy Minced Beef & Onion
     Pie Filling
Extra Hot Chicken Curry
Hamburgers with Onions &
     Gravy
Irish Stew
Minced Beef & Onion in Gravy
Prime Quality Ham

Meat Products - Frozen
Beefburgers
Economy Burgers
Faggots in Rich Sauce
Grillsteaks

Cold Meats
Bierwurst
Black Pudding Ring

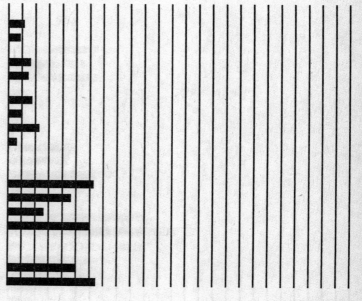

238

♦ = negligible

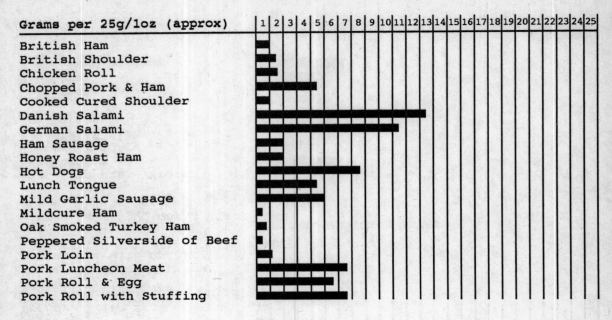

Grams per 25g/1oz (approx)	1	2	3	4	5	6	7	8	9	10	11	12	13	14	15	16	17	18	19	20	21	22	23	24	25
British Ham																									
British Shoulder																									
Chicken Roll																									
Chopped Pork & Ham																									
Cooked Cured Shoulder																									
Danish Salami																									
German Salami																									
Ham Sausage																									
Honey Roast Ham																									
Hot Dogs																									
Lunch Tongue																									
Mild Garlic Sausage																									
Mildcure Ham																									
Oak Smoked Turkey Ham																									
Peppered Silverside of Beef																									
Pork Loin																									
Pork Luncheon Meat																									
Pork Roll & Egg																									
Pork Roll with Stuffing																									

239

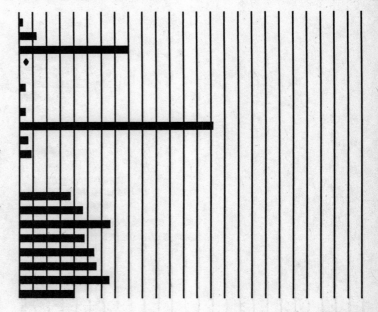

Prime Turkey	
Roast Pork	
Smoked Pork Sausage	
Smoked Turkey Breast	♦
Thin Sliced Cured Chicken Breast	
Thin Sliced Cured Turkey Breast	
Thin Sliced Danish Salami	
Thin Sliced Smoked Ham	
Thin Sliced Topside of Beef	
Sausages - Cooked	
Beef	
Butchers Choice Pork & Beef	
Cocktail	
Cumberland	
Economy	
Economy Sausagemeat (raw)	
Pork	
Pork & Beef	

♦ = negligible

240

Grams per 25g/1oz (approx)

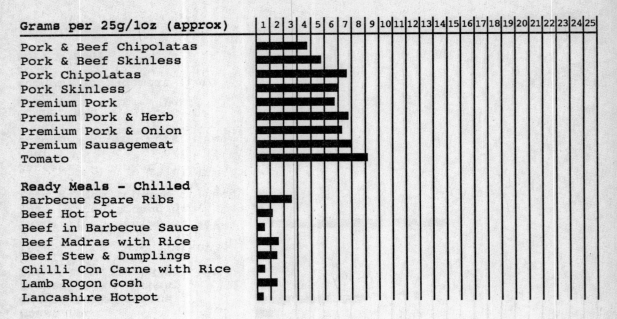

	1	2	3	4	5	6	7	8	9	10	11	12	13	14	15	16	17	18	19	20	21	22	23	24	25
Pork & Beef Chipolatas																									
Pork & Beef Skinless																									
Pork Chipolatas																									
Pork Skinless																									
Premium Pork																									
Premium Pork & Herb																									
Premium Pork & Onion																									
Premium Sausagemeat																									
Tomato																									

Ready Meals – Chilled

- Barbecue Spare Ribs
- Beef Hot Pot
- Beef in Barbecue Sauce
- Beef Madras with Rice
- Beef Stew & Dumplings
- Chilli Con Carne with Rice
- Lamb Rogon Gosh
- Lancashire Hotpot

241

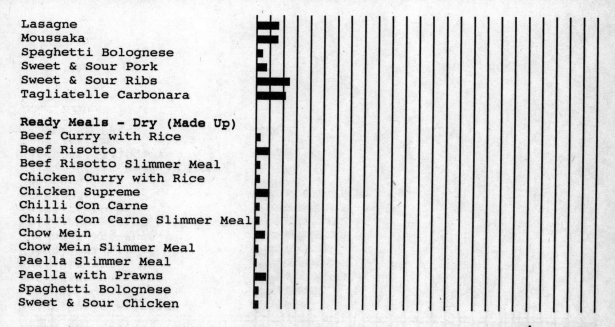

Lasagne
Moussaka
Spaghetti Bolognese
Sweet & Sour Pork
Sweet & Sour Ribs
Tagliatelle Carbonara

Ready Meals - Dry (Made Up)
Beef Curry with Rice
Beef Risotto
Beef Risotto Slimmer Meal
Chicken Curry with Rice
Chicken Supreme
Chilli Con Carne
Chilli Con Carne Slimmer Meal
Chow Mein
Chow Mein Slimmer Meal
Paella Slimmer Meal
Paella with Prawns
Spaghetti Bolognese
Sweet & Sour Chicken

◆ = negligible

Grams per 25g/1oz (approx)	1	2	3	4	5	6	7	8	9	10	11	12	13	14	15	16	17	18	19	20	21	22	23	24	25

Ready Meals - Frozen

Beef Hotpot	█																								
Beef Lasagne	█▌																								
Beef Risotto	█▌																								
Cannelloni	█▌																								
Chasseur Provencale	█																								
Chilli Con Carne with Rice	▌																								
Kashmiri Korma	█																								
Moussaka	█▌																								
Shepherds Pie	█▌																								
Sliced Roast Beef in Gravy	█																								
Spaghetti Bolognese	█																								
Tagliatelle with Ham in Cream Sauce	█▌																								

WAITROSE

243

Bacon
Danish Bacon Gammon Joint
Danish Sweet Back Bacon
Dutch Rindless Back Bacon
Dutch Middle Bacon
Half Gammon Steaks
Honey Cured Gammon Steak
Rindless Streaky Bacon
Streaky Bacon
Unsmoked Gammon Steaks
Unsmoked Back Bacon
Unsmoked Lean Back Rashers
Unsmoked Streaky Bacon

Beef
Beef Braising Steak
Beef Rolled Rib
Beef Prime Rib
Beef Stewing Steak Sliced
Beef Fillet Steak
Beef Sirloin Steaks

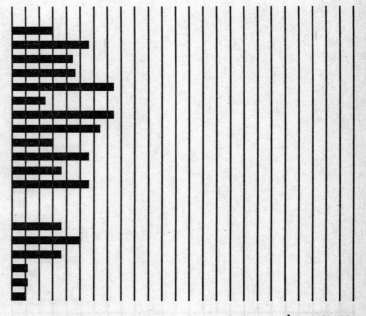

♦ = negligible

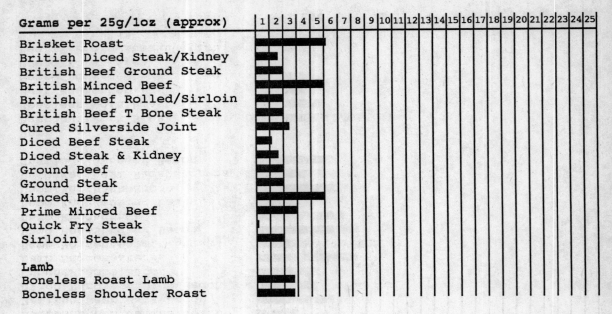

Grams per 25g/1oz (approx) 1 2 3 4 5 6 7 8 9 10 11 12 13 14 15 16 17 18 19 20 21 22 23 24 25

Brisket Roast
British Diced Steak/Kidney
British Beef Ground Steak
British Minced Beef
British Beef Rolled/Sirloin
British Beef T Bone Steak
Cured Silverside Joint
Diced Beef Steak
Diced Steak & Kidney
Ground Beef
Ground Steak
Minced Beef
Prime Minced Beef
Quick Fry Steak
Sirloin Steaks

Lamb
Boneless Roast Lamb
Boneless Shoulder Roast

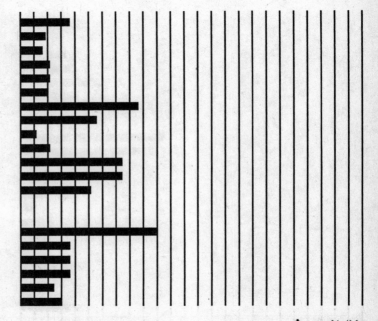

British Ground Lamb
British Lamb Kebabs
British Lamb
Diced Lamb
Ground Lamb
Lamb Leg Steak
Lamb Noisette
Lamb Roast
Lamb Brochettes
Lamb Knuckles
Lamb Shish Kebabs
Lamb Meatball Kebab
Stuffed Melon of Lamb

Pork
Barbecue Pork Ribs
Boneless Loin Roast
British Minced Pork
Cured Pork Leg
Diced Pork
Leg of Pork with Stuffing

♦ = negligible

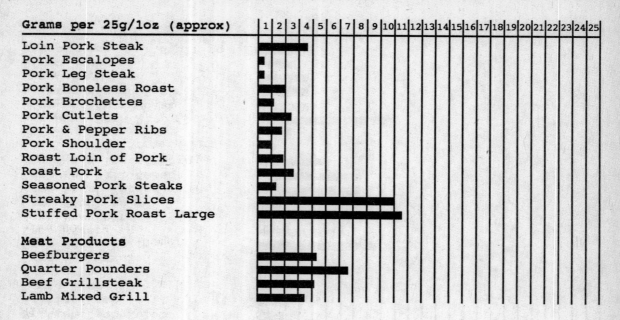

Grams per 25g/1oz (approx)	1	2	3	4	5	6	7	8	9	10	11	12	13	14	15	16	17	18	19	20	21	22	23	24	25
Loin Pork Steak																									
Pork Escalopes																									
Pork Leg Steak																									
Pork Boneless Roast																									
Pork Brochettes																									
Pork Cutlets																									
Pork & Pepper Ribs																									
Pork Shoulder																									
Roast Loin of Pork																									
Roast Pork																									
Seasoned Pork Steaks																									
Streaky Pork Slices																									
Stuffed Pork Roast Large																									

Meat Products

	1	2	3	4	5	6	7	8	9	10	11	12	13	14	15	16	17	18	19	20	21	22	23	24	25
Beefburgers																									
Quarter Pounders																									
Beef Grillsteak																									
Lamb Mixed Grill																									

Veal Escalope
Minced Lamb Grill
Yorkshire Fry
Rabbit Casserole Pieces

Ready Meals
Beef Stew with Dumplings
Biks Beef Hash
Chilli Con Carne
Lamb Boulangere
Lamb Curry
Lamb Rogan Josh
Lasagne
Leek, Bacon & Tomato Savoury
Moussaka (Frozen)
Moussaka
Potato, Onion & Ham Bake
Prawn Curry
Savoury Supper
Shepherds Pie
Somerset Supper

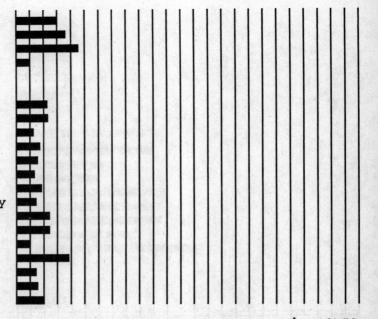

♦ = negligible

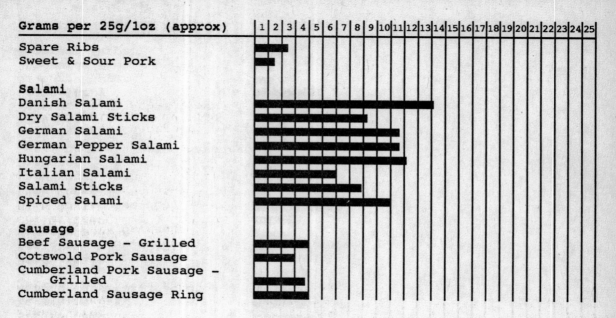

Grams per 25g/1oz (approx)	1	2	3	4	5	6	7	8	9	10	11	12	13	14	15	16	17	18	19	20	21	22	23	24	25
Spare Ribs																									
Sweet & Sour Pork																									
Salami																									
Danish Salami																									
Dry Salami Sticks																									
German Salami																									
German Pepper Salami																									
Hungarian Salami																									
Italian Salami																									
Salami Sticks																									
Spiced Salami																									
Sausage																									
Beef Sausage – Grilled																									
Cotswold Pork Sausage																									
Cumberland Pork Sausage – Grilled																									
Cumberland Sausage Ring																									

249

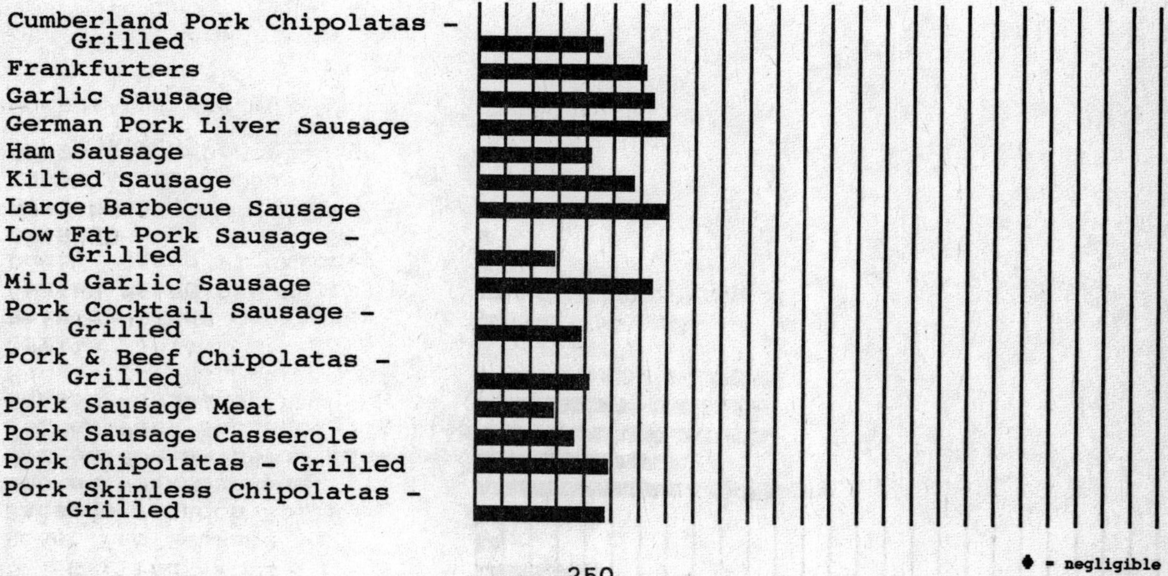

Food	
Cumberland Pork Chipolatas – Grilled	
Frankfurters	
Garlic Sausage	
German Pork Liver Sausage	
Ham Sausage	
Kilted Sausage	
Large Barbecue Sausage	
Low Fat Pork Sausage – Grilled	
Mild Garlic Sausage	
Pork Cocktail Sausage – Grilled	
Pork & Beef Chipolatas – Grilled	
Pork Sausage Meat	
Pork Sausage Casserole	
Pork Chipolatas – Grilled	
Pork Skinless Chipolatas – Grilled	

250

♦ = negligible

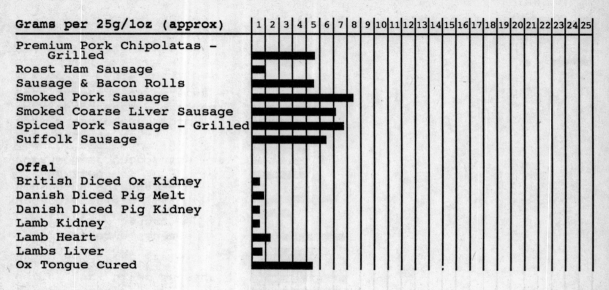

Grams per 25g/1oz (approx)	1	2	3	4	5	6	7	8	9	10	11	12	13	14	15	16	17	18	19	20	21	22	23	24	25
Premium Pork Chipolatas – Grilled					5																				
Roast Ham Sausage		2																							
Sausage & Bacon Rolls					5																				
Smoked Pork Sausage							8																		
Smoked Coarse Liver Sausage						7																			
Spiced Pork Sausage – Grilled							7																		
Suffolk Sausage						6																			

Offal

	1	2	3	4	5	6	7	8	9	10	11	12	13	14	15	16	17	18	19	20	21	22	23	24	25
British Diced Ox Kidney	1																								
Danish Diced Pig Melt	1																								
Danish Diced Pig Kidney	1																								
Lamb Kidney	1																								
Lamb Heart		2																							
Lambs Liver	1																								
Ox Tongue Cured					5																				

Cold Meats

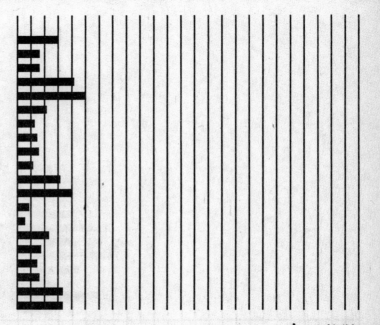

Apricot Mini Ham
Baked Gammon Roll
Beechwood Smoked Ham
Boneless Ham
Brawn Hungarian Style
Brawn
Buckingham Ham
Continental Honey Roast Ham
Cooked Brisket
Cooked Cured Shoulder
Corned Beef
Cured Ox Tongue
French Country Ham
Ham
Haslet
Honey Roast Ham
Maryland Ham
Mustard & Honey Roast Ham
Oak Smoked English Ham
Old English Virginia Ham

♦ = negligible

Grams per 25g/1oz (approx)	1	2	3	4	5	6	7	8	9	10	11	12	13	14	15	16	17	18	19	20	21	22	23	24	25
Peppered Ham																									
Pork/Beef Luncheon Meat																									
Pork Tongue																									
Roast Mini Ham																									
Roast Pork Loin																									
Roast Topside of Beef																									
Roast Beef																									
Shoulder																									
Smoked Ham																									
Spiced Ham																									
Traditional Matured York Ham																									

MILK & CREAM PRODUCTS & SUBSTITUTES - GENERAL

Milk, Cow's:
Channel Isles
Condensed, Skimmed
Condensed, Whole

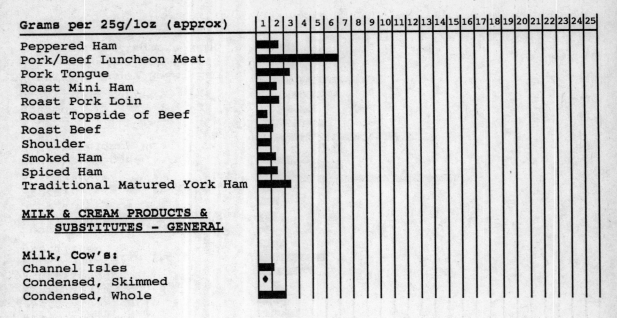

253

Dried, Whole
Dried, Skimmed
Evaporated, Whole
Fresh, Skimmed
Fresh, Whole
Longlife, UHT
Sterilised

Milk, Goats

Cream:
Cornish Clotted
Diet Double
Diet Single
Double
Single
Soured
Sterilised Canned
Whipping

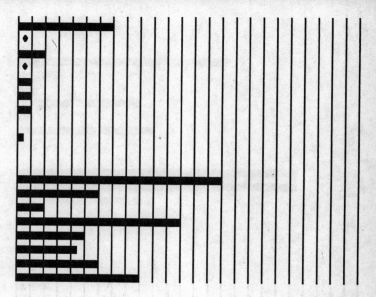

254

♦ = negligible

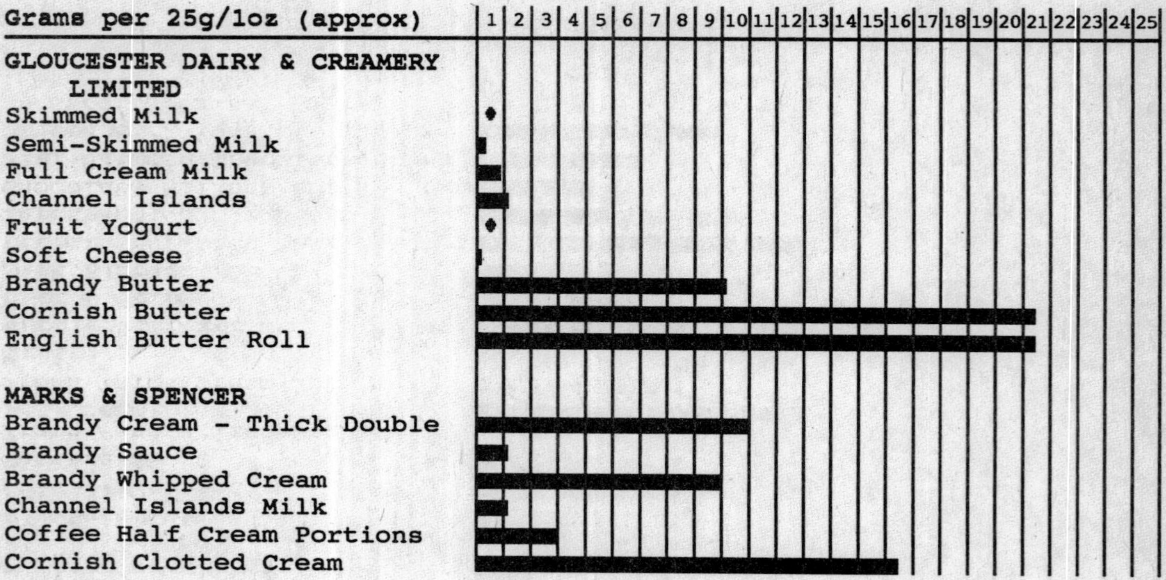
Grams per 25g/1oz (approx)
1 2 3 4 5 6 7 8 9 10 11 12 13 14 15 16 17 18 19 20 21 22 23 24 25
GLOUCESTER DAIRY & CREAMERY LIMITED
Skimmed Milk
Semi-Skimmed Milk
Full Cream Milk
Channel Islands
Fruit Yogurt
Soft Cheese
Brandy Butter
Cornish Butter
English Butter Roll
MARKS & SPENCER
Brandy Cream - Thick Double
Brandy Sauce
Brandy Whipped Cream
Channel Islands Milk
Coffee Half Cream Portions
Cornish Clotted Cream

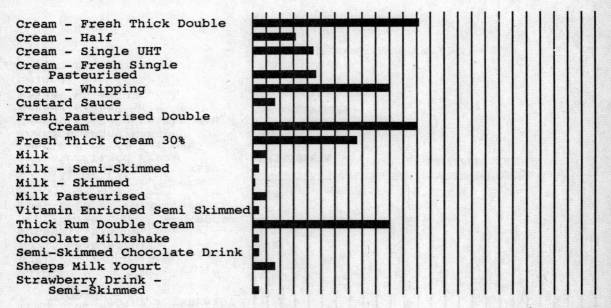

Cream – Fresh Thick Double	
Cream – Half	
Cream – Single UHT	
Cream – Fresh Single Pasteurised	
Cream – Whipping	
Custard Sauce	
Fresh Pasteurised Double Cream	
Fresh Thick Cream 30%	
Milk	
Milk – Semi-Skimmed	
Milk – Skimmed	
Milk Pasteurised	
Vitamin Enriched Semi Skimmed	
Thick Rum Double Cream	
Chocolate Milkshake	
Semi-Skimmed Chocolate Drink	
Sheeps Milk Yogurt	
Strawberry Drink – Semi-Skimmed	

♦ = negligible

256

Grams per 25g/1oz (approx)	1	2	3	4	5	6	7	8	9	10	11	12	13	14	15	16	17	18	19	20	21	22	23	24	25

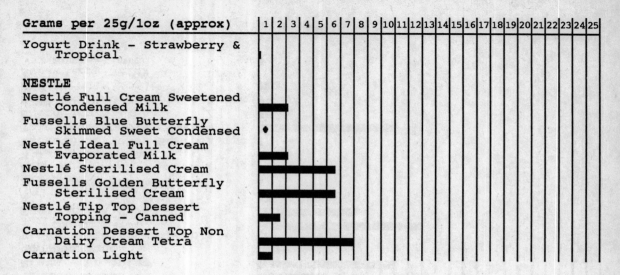

Yogurt Drink - Strawberry & Tropical

NESTLE

Nestlé Full Cream Sweetened Condensed Milk

Fussells Blue Butterfly Skimmed Sweet Condensed

Nestlé Ideal Full Cream Evaporated Milk

Nestlé Sterilised Cream

Fussells Golden Butterfly Sterilised Cream

Nestlé Tip Top Dessert Topping - Canned

Carnation Dessert Top Non Dairy Cream Tetra

Carnation Light

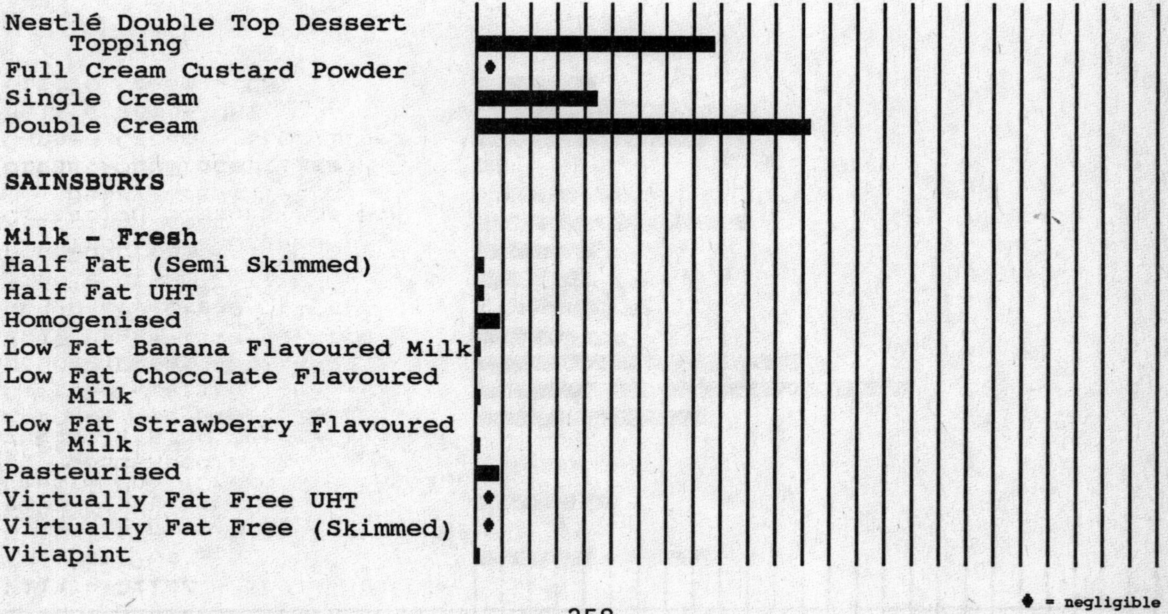

Nestlé Double Top Dessert Topping	
Full Cream Custard Powder	
Single Cream	
Double Cream	

SAINSBURYS

Milk - Fresh
Half Fat (Semi Skimmed)
Half Fat UHT
Homogenised
Low Fat Banana Flavoured Milk
Low Fat Chocolate Flavoured Milk
Low Fat Strawberry Flavoured Milk
Pasteurised
Virtually Fat Free UHT
Virtually Fat Free (Skimmed)
Vitapint

◆ = negligible

258

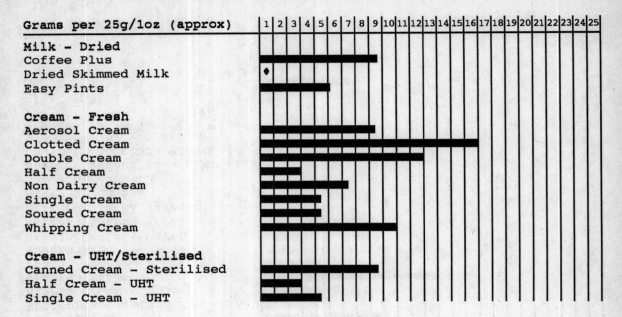

Grams per 25g/1oz (approx)	1	2	3	4	5	6	7	8	9	10	11	12	13	14	15	16	17	18	19	20	21	22	23	24	25

Milk - Dried
Coffee Plus
Dried Skimmed Milk
Easy Pints

Cream - Fresh
Aerosol Cream
Clotted Cream
Double Cream
Half Cream
Non Dairy Cream
Single Cream
Soured Cream
Whipping Cream

Cream - UHT/Sterilised
Canned Cream - Sterilised
Half Cream - UHT
Single Cream - UHT

259

ST IVEL
Fresh Cream
Single Cream
Whipping Cream
Clotted Cream
Soured Cream
Double Cream – UHT
Single Cream – UHT
Whipping Cream – UHT

TESCO

Milk – Fresh
Whole
Semi-skimmed
Skimmed

Milk – Dried
Makes 5 Pints
Skimmed

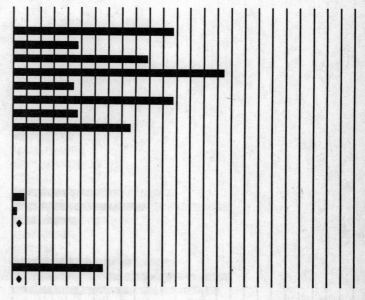

♦ = negligible

Grams per 25g/1oz (approx)	1	2	3	4	5	6	7	8	9	10	11	12	13	14	15	16	17	18	19	20	21	22	23	24	25

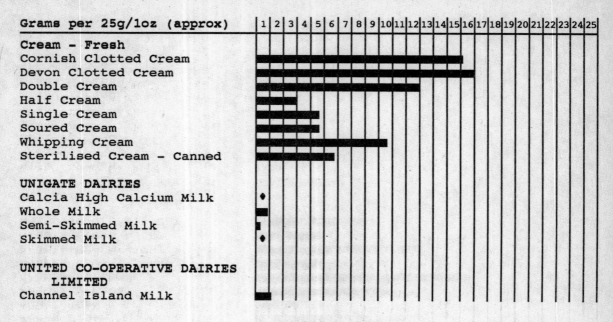

Cream - Fresh
Cornish Clotted Cream
Devon Clotted Cream
Double Cream
Half Cream
Single Cream
Soured Cream
Whipping Cream
Sterilised Cream - Canned

UNIGATE DAIRIES
Calcia High Calcium Milk
Whole Milk
Semi-Skimmed Milk
Skimmed Milk

UNITED CO-OPERATIVE DAIRIES
    LIMITED
Channel Island Milk

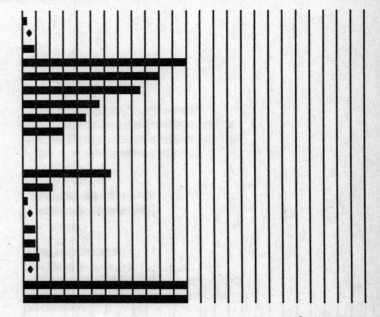

Semi-Skimmed Milk	
Skimmed Milk	♦
Whole Milk	
Double Cream	
Whipping Cream	
Whipping Cream Less Fat	
Sterilised Cream	
Single Cream	
Half Cream	
WAITROSE	
Skimmed Milk/Veg Fat	
Evaporated Milk	
Semi-Skimmed Milk - UHT	
Skimmed Milk - UHT	♦
Full Cream Milk - UHT	
Full Cream Milk	
Channel Isle Milk	
Fresh Skimmed Milk	♦
Extra Thick Double Cream	
Fresh Double Cream	

♦ = negligible

262

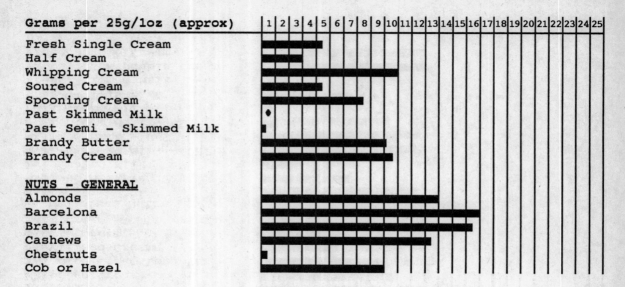

Grams per 25g/1oz (approx)	1	2	3	4	5	6	7	8	9	10	11	12	13	14	15	16	17	18	19	20	21	22	23	24	25
Fresh Single Cream																									
Half Cream																									
Whipping Cream																									
Soured Cream																									
Spooning Cream																									
Past Skimmed Milk																									
Past Semi - Skimmed Milk																									
Brandy Butter																									
Brandy Cream																									

NUTS - GENERAL

Almonds																									
Barcelona																									
Brazil																									
Cashews																									
Chestnuts																									
Cob or Hazel																									

263

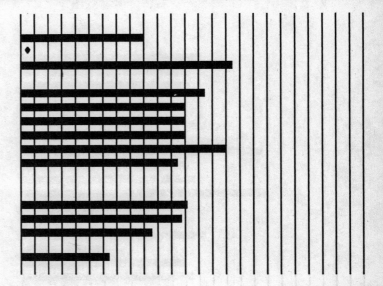

Coconut:
Fresh
Milk ◆
Desiccated

Peanuts:
Dry Roasted
Fresh
Roasted & Salted
Peanut Butter
Salted Mixed Nuts
Walnuts

KP
Roast Salted Peanuts
Roast Salted Cashews
Mixed Nuts & Raisins
Trebles (Nuts, Raisins &
    Choc Chips)

◆ = negligible

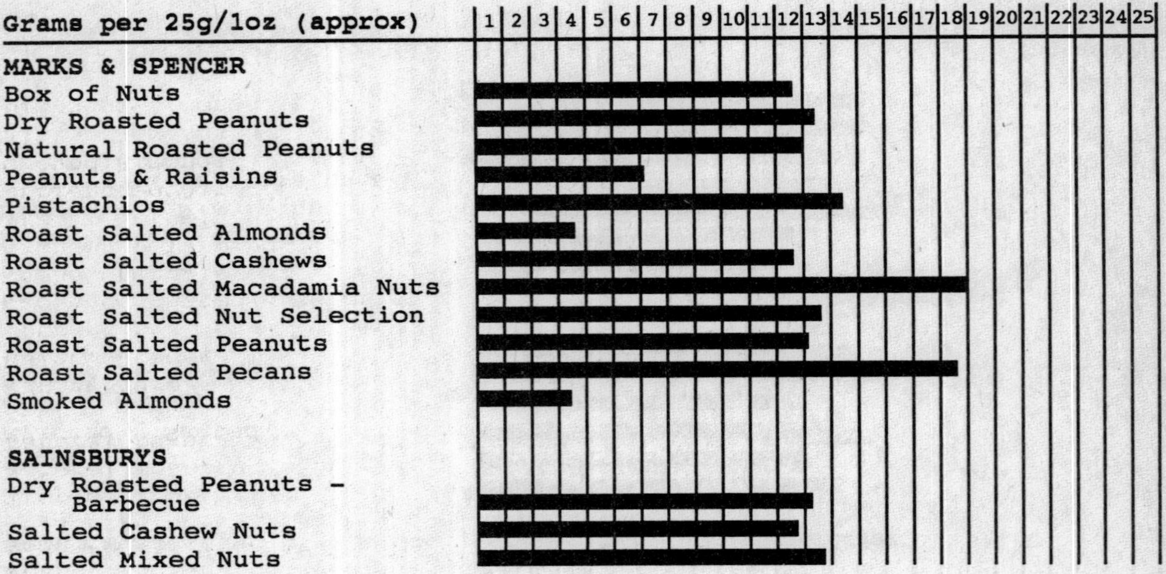

Grams per 25g/1oz (approx) — scale: 1 2 3 4 5 6 7 8 9 10 11 12 13 14 15 16 17 18 19 20 21 22 23 24 25

MARKS & SPENCER

Item	Grams per 25g/1oz (approx)
Box of Nuts	12
Dry Roasted Peanuts	13
Natural Roasted Peanuts	11½
Peanuts & Raisins	6½
Pistachios	14
Roast Salted Almonds	4
Roast Salted Cashews	12
Roast Salted Macadamia Nuts	19
Roast Salted Nut Selection	13½
Roast Salted Peanuts	13
Roast Salted Pecans	18½
Smoked Almonds	4

SAINSBURYS

Item	Grams per 25g/1oz (approx)
Dry Roasted Peanuts – Barbecue	13
Salted Cashew Nuts	12½
Salted Mixed Nuts	14

265

Salted Peanuts
Peanut Kernels
Peanuts & Raisins
Peanuts, Raisins & Milk Choc
    Chips
Tropical Nut Mix
Natural Roasted Peanuts
Natural Luxury Nut Selection

Baking Nuts
Walnut Pieces
Chopped Mix Nuts
Chopped Roasted Hazelnuts
Cashew Kernels
Crunchnut Topping
Brazil Kernels
Unblanched Almonds
Ground Almonds
Flaked Almonds
Blanched Almonds

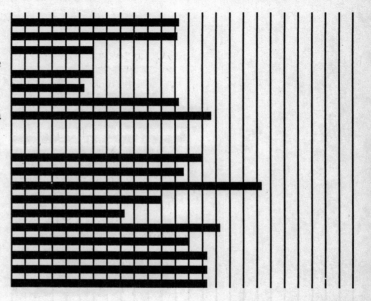

266

♦ = negligible

Grams per 25g/1oz (approx)	Value
TESCO	
Bombay Mix	7
Cashew Nuts	11
Dry Roasted Peanuts	13
Exotic Fruit & Nut Mix	7
Honey Coated Peanuts	10
Light Peanuts	12
Mixed Nuts & Raisins	7
Monkey Nuts (Shelled)	13
Nuts, Raisins & Choc Chips	8
Peanut Kernels	13
Roasted Mixed Nuts & Raisins	11
Roasted Salted Peanuts	13
Salted Cashew Nuts	13
Salted Mixed Nuts	14
Sesame Nut Crunch	11
Yogurt Raisins	6

267

WAITROSE
Almonds Hick Smoked
Caribbean Mix
Dry Roasted Peanuts
Fruit, Nuts & Seeds
Lightly Salted Peanuts
Lower Fat Large Peanuts
Mixed Nuts & Raisins
Pistachio Nuts
Roast Salted Peanuts
Salted Cashews
Salted Mixed Nuts
Salted Large Peanuts
Tropical Fruit & Nuts
Yogurt Coated Nuts & Raisins

<u>PANCAKES</u>

MARKS & SPENCER
Sultana and Syrup Pancakes

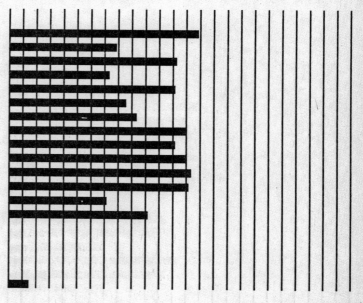

◆ = negligible

Grams per 25g/1oz (approx)	1	2	3	4	5	6	7	8	9	10	11	12	13	14	15	16	17	18	19	20	21	22	23	24	25

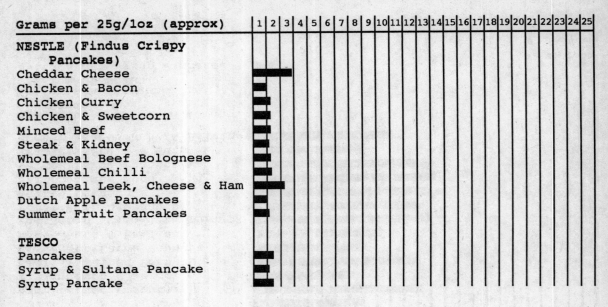

NESTLE (Findus Crispy Pancakes)

Cheddar Cheese

Chicken & Bacon

Chicken Curry

Chicken & Sweetcorn

Minced Beef

Steak & Kidney

Wholemeal Beef Bolognese

Wholemeal Chilli

Wholemeal Leek, Cheese & Ham

Dutch Apple Pancakes

Summer Fruit Pancakes

TESCO

Pancakes

Syrup & Sultana Pancake

Syrup Pancake

WAITROSE
Mexican Pancakes

PASTA & PASTA PRODUCTS -
        GENERAL
Lasagne
Macaroni
Spaghetti, Boiled
Spaghetti, Canned in Tomato
        Sauce
Tagliatelle

CO-OP
Spaghetti in Tomato Sauce
Spaghetti Rings in Tomato
        Sauce
Spaghetti Numbers in Tomato
        Sauce
Wholewheat Spaghetti in
        Tomato Sauce

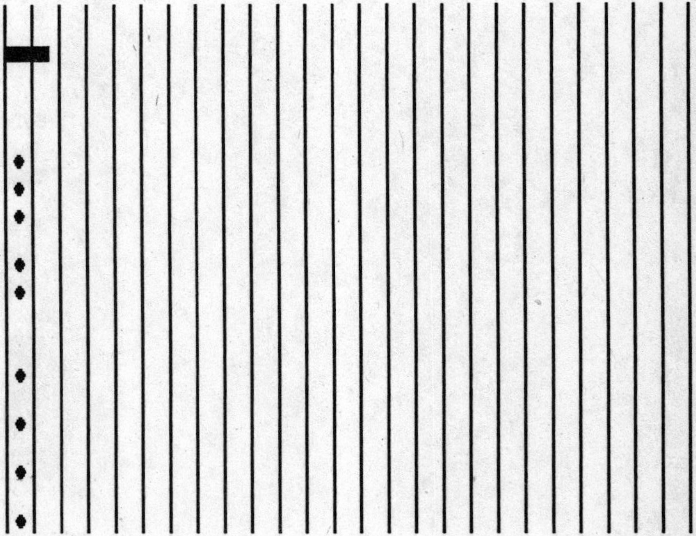

◆ = negligible

270

Grams per 25g/1oz (approx)	1	2	3	4	5	6	7	8	9	10	11	12	13	14	15	16	17	18	19	20	21	22	23	24	25
Spaghetti in Reduced Sugar & Salt Tomato Sauce	◆																								
HEINZ																									
Haunted House – Spaghetti Shapes in Tomato Sauce	◆																								
Invaders – Spaghetti Shapes in Tomato Sauce	◆																								
Invaders with Meateors	▮																								
Macaroni Cheese	▬																								
Noodle Doodles	◆																								
Ravioli in Beef & Tomato Sauce	▮																								
Ravioli in Tomato Sauce	▮																								
Spaghetti Bolognese	▬																								
Spaghetti Hoops in Tomato Sauce	◆																								
Spaghetti in Tomato Sauce	◆																								

Wholewheat Pasta Shells in
    Spicy Tomato Sauce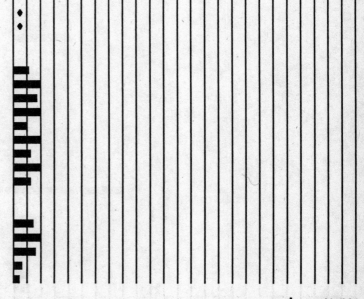
Wholewheat Spaghetti

ICELAND
Cannelloni
Fettucini
Lasagne
Lasagne Verdi
Moussaka
Spaghetti Bolognese
Tagliatelle
Tortellini
Vegetable Lasagne

MARKS & SPENCER
Cannelloni
Lasagne
Lasagne - Fresh
Lasagne Pasta
Minestrone Soup

272

♦ = negligible

Grams per 25g/1oz (approx)	1	2	3	4	5	6	7	8	9	10	11	12	13	14	15	16	17	18	19	20	21	22	23	24	25
Ravioli																									
Spaghetti Bolognese – Frozen																									
Spaghetti																									
Tagliatelle																									
Tagliatelle – Green																									
Tagliatelle – New Style																									
Tagliatelle – White																									
Tagliatelle – with Vegetables																									
NESTLE																									
Findus Lean Cuisine																									
Lasagne Verdi																									
Spaghetti Bolognese																									
Zucchini Lasagne																									
Crosse & Blackwell – Pasta Choice																									
A La Creme																									

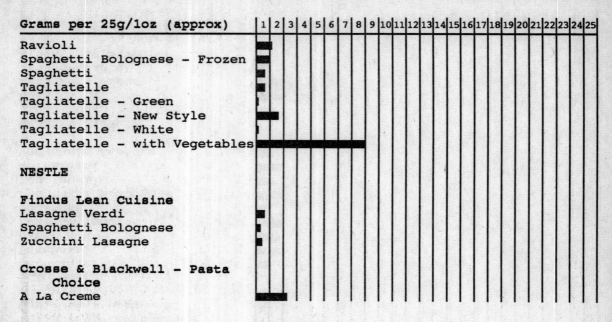

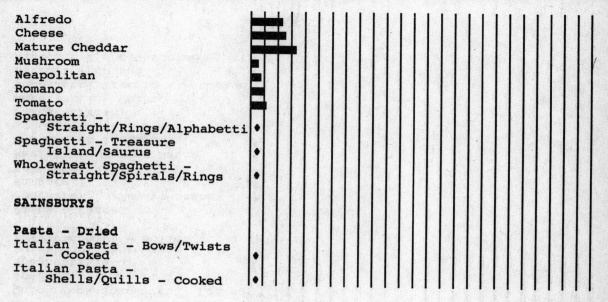

Alfredo
Cheese
Mature Cheddar
Mushroom
Neapolitan
Romano
Tomato
Spaghetti –
    Straight/Rings/Alphabetti
Spaghetti – Treasure
    Island/Saurus
Wholewheat Spaghetti –
    Straight/Spirals/Rings

SAINSBURYS

Pasta – Dried
Italian Pasta – Bows/Twists
    – Cooked
Italian Pasta –
    Shells/Quills – Cooked

♦ = negligible

Grams per 25g/1oz (approx)	1	2	3	4	5	6	7	8	9	10	11	12	13	14	15	16	17	18	19	20	21	22	23	24	25
Macaroni	♦																								
Quick Cook Spaghetti - Boiled	▌																								
Spaghetti - Boiled	▌																								
Spaghetti Verdi	■																								
Quick Cook Wholewheat Spaghetti - Boiled	▌																								
Pasta - Canned																									
Spaghetti in Tomato Sauce	♦																								
Numberelli	♦																								
Spaghetti Rings	♦																								
Ravioli in Tomato Sauce	♦																								
Wholewheat Spaghetti	♦																								
Pasta - Fresh																									
Capelletti - Cooked	■																								
Capelletti Trecolori - Cooked	■																								
Ravioli - Cooked	■																								
Paglia e Fieno - Cooked	♦																								

275

Tagliatelle – Cooked	◆
Tagliatelle Verdi – Cooked	◆
Tortellini Spinach – Cooked	▪
Ready Meals – Frozen	
Cannelloni	
Cannelloni Verdi	
Kedgeree	
Lasagne	
Lasagne Pescatore (Chilled)	
Lasagne Verdi	
Tagliatelle with Ham & Mushrooms	
TESCO	
Spaghetti in Tomato Sauce (all shapes) – Canned	◆
Egg Tagliatelle Verdi	◆
Pasta – Bows/Couches/Quills	◆
Pasta – Shells/Twists/Wheels	◆
Quick Cook Egg Lasagne	◆

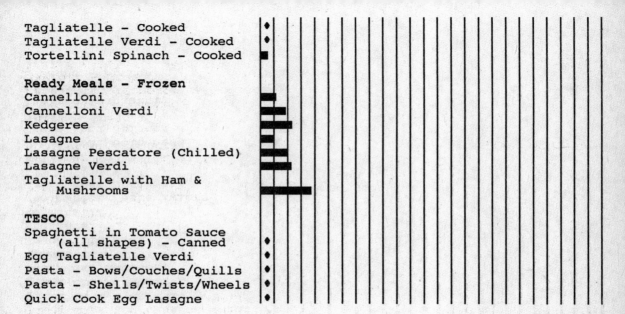

276

◆ = negligible

Grams per 25g/1oz (approx)	1	2	3	4	5	6	7	8	9	10	11	12	13	14	15	16	17	18	19	20	21	22	23	24	25
Quick Cook Egg Lasagne Verdi	♦																								
Quick Cook Macaroni	♦																								
Quick Cook Spaghetti	♦																								
Short Cut Macaroni	♦																								
Spaghetti	♦																								
Spaghetti Verdi	♦																								
Tagliatelle	♦																								
Vermicelli	♦																								
Wholewheat Pasta Twists	▌																								
Wholewheat Spaghetti	▌																								
WAITROSE																									
Cannelloni Bolognese	██																								
Cannelloni Spinach	███																								
Capellini	▌																								
Italian Spaghetti	▌																								
Lasagne	██																								
Lasagne - Frozen	██																								
Macaroni	▌																								

277

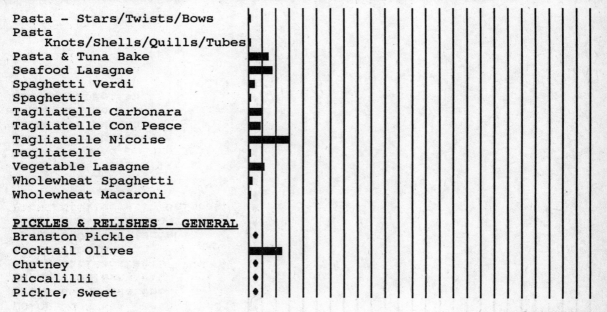

Pasta - Stars/Twists/Bows	
Pasta Knots/Shells/Quills/Tubes	
Pasta & Tuna Bake	
Seafood Lasagne	
Spaghetti Verdi	
Spaghetti	
Tagliatelle Carbonara	
Tagliatelle Con Pesce	
Tagliatelle Nicoise	
Tagliatelle	
Vegetable Lasagne	
Wholewheat Spaghetti	
Wholewheat Macaroni	

PICKLES & RELISHES - GENERAL

Branston Pickle	◆
Cocktail Olives	
Chutney	◆
Piccalilli	◆
Pickle, Sweet	◆

◆ = negligible

Grams per 25g/1oz (approx)	1	2	3	4	5	6	7	8	9	10	11	12	13	14	15	16	17	18	19	20	21	22	23	24	25
CO-OP																									
Crinkle Cut Beetroot	•																								
Mixed Pickles	•																								
Piccalilli	▍																								
Pickled Onions	•																								
Pickled Onions (Brown)	•																								
Pickled Red Cabbage	•																								
Pickled Silverskin Onions	•																								
Sliced Beetroot	•																								
Sweet Pickle	•																								
Sweetened Piccalilli	▍																								
Sweet Pickled Onions	•																								
Whole Baby Beetroots	•																								
Hamburger Relish	•																								
Onion Relish	•																								
Sweetcorn Relish	•																								

HEINZ
Ploughmans Mild Mustard
    Pickle
Ploughmans Pickle
Ploughmans Tomato Pickle

NESTLE (Crosse & Blackwell)
Branston Pickle
Branston Sandwich Pickle

RHM GROCERY (SHARWOODS)
American Barbecue Quick
    Marinade
Apricot Chutney
Bengal Hot Mango Chutney
Curried Fruit Chutney
Green Label Mango Chutney
Mango & Apple Chutney
Peach Chutney
Special Vegetable Chutney
Tomato & Courgette Chutney

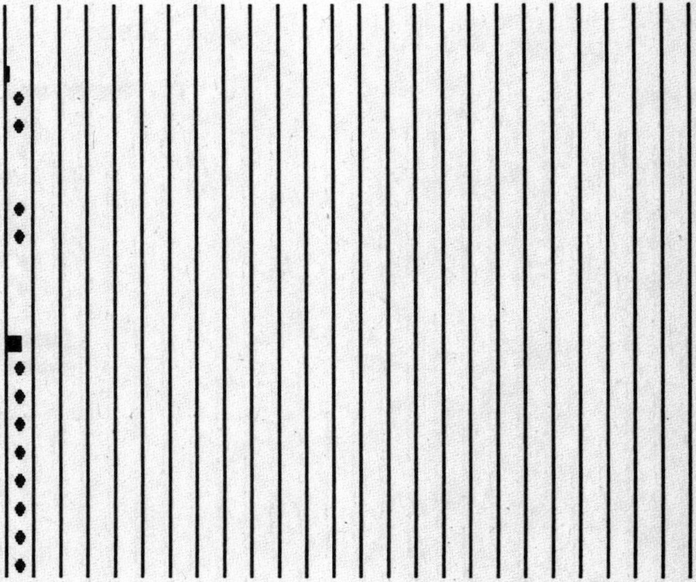

♦ = negligible

280

Grams per 25g/1oz (approx)	1	2	3	4	5	6	7	8	9	10	11	12	13	14	15	16	17	18	19	20	21	22	23	24	25
SAINSBURYS																									
Barbecue Relish	◆																								
Cider Vinegar	◆																								
Cocktail Cherries	◆																								
Corn Relish	◆																								
Courgette Chutney	◆																								
Cucumber Relish	◆																								
Curried Fruit Chutney	◆																								
Dijon Mustard	■	■																							
English Mustard	■	■																							
Malt Vinegar	◆																								
Midget Gherkins	◆																								
Mild Mustard Relish	◆																								
Mustard with Herbs	■																								
Onion Relish	◆																								
Piccalilli	◆																								
Pickled Onions	◆																								
Pickled Red Cabbage	◆																								
Pitted Black Olives	■	■	■	■	■																				

Red Wine Vinegar
Shredded Beetroot in Sweet
    Vinegar
Silverskin Onions
Sweet Onions
Sweet Piccalilli
Tomato Relish
Tomato & Chilli Relish
Vinegar – White Wine
Whole Baby Beets

TESCO
Apricot Chutney
Beansprout Salad
Beetroot in Sweet Vinegar
Cocktail Gherkins
Cocktail Olives
Cocktail Onions
Continental Style Mixed
    Pickle
Curried Fruit Chutney

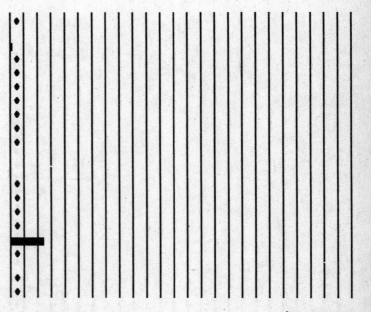

♦ = negligible

Grams per 25g/1oz (approx)	1	2	3	4	5	6	7	8	9	10	11	12	13	14	15	16	17	18	19	20	21	22	23	24	25
Peach Chutney	♦																								
Piccalilli	♦																								
Pickled Beetroot	♦																								
Pickled Cucumber	♦																								
Pickled Onions	♦																								
Pickled Red Cabbage	♦																								
Pickled Silverskin Onions	♦																								
Sweet Piccalilli	♦																								
Sweet Pickle	♦																								
Sweet Pickled Onions	♦																								
Mild Mustard Relish	♦																								
Onion Relish	♦																								
Sweetcorn Relish	♦																								
Tomato Relish	♦																								
Tomato and Chilli Relish	♦																								
WAITROSE																									
Apple/Sultana Chutney	♦																								
Apple/Onion Chutney	♦																								

```
Apricot/Ginger Chutney        ♦ |  |  |  |  |  |  |  |  |  |  |  |  |  |  |  |  |  |  |  |
Cocktail Onions               ♦ |  |  |  |  |  |  |  |  |  |  |  |  |  |  |  |  |  |  |  |
Cocktail Gherkins             ♦ |  |  |  |  |  |  |  |  |  |  |  |  |  |  |  |  |  |  |  |
Curry Chutney                 ♦ |  |  |  |  |  |  |  |  |  |  |  |  |  |  |  |  |  |  |  |
Gherkins                      ♦ |  |  |  |  |  |  |  |  |  |  |  |  |  |  |  |  |  |  |  |
Mango Chutney                 ♦ |  |  |  |  |  |  |  |  |  |  |  |  |  |  |  |  |  |  |  |
Mixed Pickles In Vinegar      ♦ |  |  |  |  |  |  |  |  |  |  |  |  |  |  |  |  |  |  |  |
Mustard Piccalilli            ♦ |  |  |  |  |  |  |  |  |  |  |  |  |  |  |  |  |  |  |  |
Peach Chutney                 ♦ |  |  |  |  |  |  |  |  |  |  |  |  |  |  |  |  |  |  |  |
Piccalilli                    ♦ |  |  |  |  |  |  |  |  |  |  |  |  |  |  |  |  |  |  |  |
Pickled Onions                ♦ |  |  |  |  |  |  |  |  |  |  |  |  |  |  |  |  |  |  |  |
Red Cabbage                   ♦ |  |  |  |  |  |  |  |  |  |  |  |  |  |  |  |  |  |  |  |
Sliced Beetroot/Vinegar       ♦ |  |  |  |  |  |  |  |  |  |  |  |  |  |  |  |  |  |  |  |
Sliced Beets                  ♦ |  |  |  |  |  |  |  |  |  |  |  |  |  |  |  |  |  |  |  |
Sweet Pickle                  ♦ |  |  |  |  |  |  |  |  |  |  |  |  |  |  |  |  |  |  |  |
Sweet Pickled Onions          ♦ |  |  |  |  |  |  |  |  |  |  |  |  |  |  |  |  |  |  |  |
Sweet Piccalilli              ♦ |  |  |  |  |  |  |  |  |  |  |  |  |  |  |  |  |  |  |  |
Tomato Chutney                ♦ |  |  |  |  |  |  |  |  |  |  |  |  |  |  |  |  |  |  |  |
```

♦ = negligible

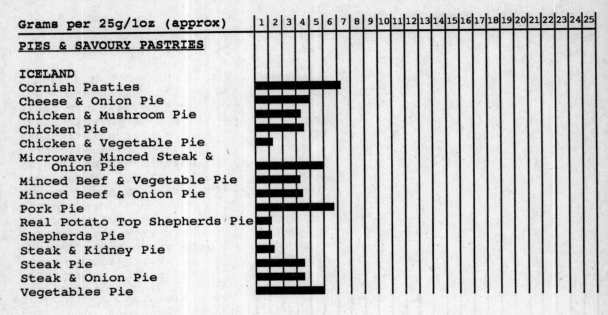

Grams per 25g/1oz (approx) |1|2|3|4|5|6|7|8|9|10|11|12|13|14|15|16|17|18|19|20|21|22|23|24|25|

PIES & SAVOURY PASTRIES

ICELAND
Cornish Pasties
Cheese & Onion Pie
Chicken & Mushroom Pie
Chicken Pie
Chicken & Vegetable Pie
Microwave Minced Steak & Onion Pie
Minced Beef & Vegetable Pie
Minced Beef & Onion Pie
Pork Pie
Real Potato Top Shepherds Pie
Shepherds Pie
Steak & Kidney Pie
Steak Pie
Steak & Onion Pie
Vegetables Pie

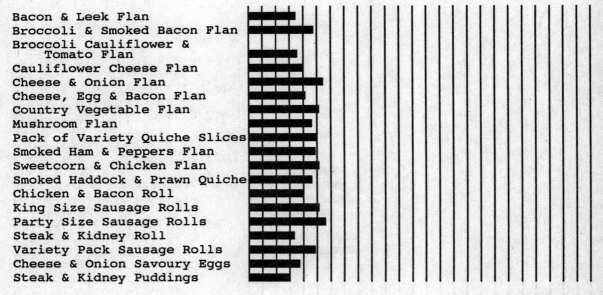

Bacon & Leek Flan
Broccoli & Smoked Bacon Flan
Broccoli Cauliflower &
    Tomato Flan
Cauliflower Cheese Flan
Cheese & Onion Flan
Cheese, Egg & Bacon Flan
Country Vegetable Flan
Mushroom Flan
Pack of Variety Quiche Slices
Smoked Ham & Peppers Flan
Sweetcorn & Chicken Flan
Smoked Haddock & Prawn Quiche
Chicken & Bacon Roll
King Size Sausage Rolls
Party Size Sausage Rolls
Steak & Kidney Roll
Variety Pack Sausage Rolls
Cheese & Onion Savoury Eggs
Steak & Kidney Puddings

♣ = negligible

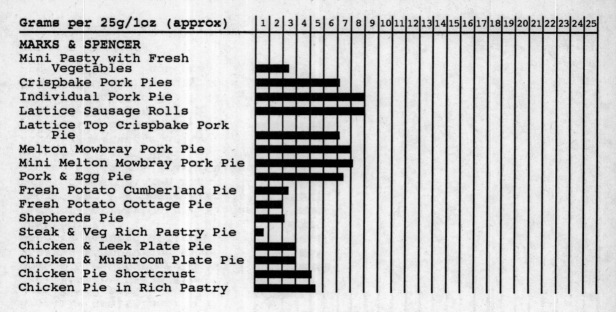

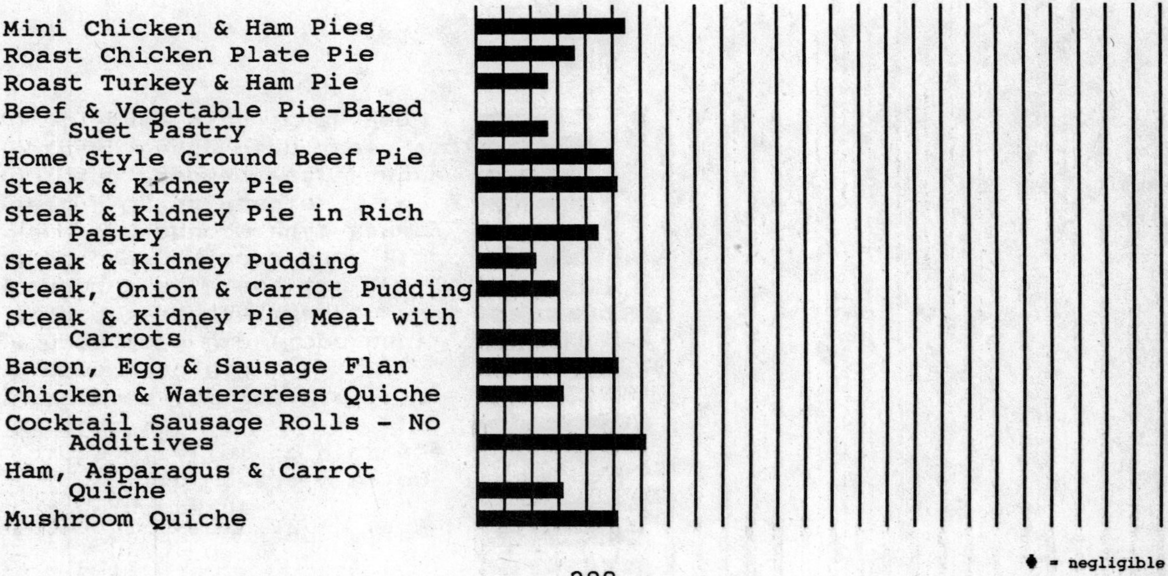

Mini Chicken & Ham Pies

Roast Chicken Plate Pie

Roast Turkey & Ham Pie

Beef & Vegetable Pie-Baked
  Suet Pastry

Home Style Ground Beef Pie

Steak & Kidney Pie

Steak & Kidney Pie in Rich
  Pastry

Steak & Kidney Pudding

Steak, Onion & Carrot Pudding

Steak & Kidney Pie Meal with
  Carrots

Bacon, Egg & Sausage Flan

Chicken & Watercress Quiche

Cocktail Sausage Rolls - No
  Additives

Ham, Asparagus & Carrot
  Quiche

Mushroom Quiche

288

♦ = negligible

Grams per 25g/1oz (approx)	1	2	3	4	5	6	7	8	9	10	11	12	13	14	15	16	17	18	19	20	21	22	23	24	25
Pork, Beef & Onion Sausage Roll	▇	▇	▇	▇	▇	▇	▇																		
Puff Pastry Sausage Rolls	▇	▇	▇	▇	▇	▇	▇																		
Quiche Lorraine	▇	▇	▇	▇	▇																				
Quiche with Cheese & Onion	▇	▇	▇	▇	▇																				
Quiche with Tomato & Cheese	▇	▇	▇	▇	▇	▇																			
Scotch Pie	▇	▇	▇	▇	▇	▇																			
Bolognese Lattice Pie	▇	▇	▇	▇	▇																				
Minced Beef Pie	▇	▇	▇	▇	▇																				
Minced Beef Pie (Topcrust)	▇	▇	▇	▇	▇																				
Minced Beef Pie Trad	▇	▇	▇	▇	▇	▇	▇																		
Minced Beef Plate Pie	▇	▇	▇	▇	▇																				
Shortcrust Minced Beef Pie	▇	▇	▇	▇	▇																				
Beef & Mushroom Puff Pastry	▇	▇																							
Beef & Onion Pasties	▇	▇	▇	▇	▇																				
Cornish Pasties Puff Pastry	▇	▇	▇																						
Cornish Pasty with Fresh Veg	▇	▇	▇																						
Mini Pasty with Fresh Veg	▇	▇	▇																						

NESTLE (Findus)
Quiche Lorraine
Tarte Aux Champignons
Tarte L'Oignon
Tart Soufflé au Fromage

SAINSBURYS
Minced Beef & Onion Pie
Beef & Onion Pasties
Beef & Vegetable Pasties
Cornish Pasty
Fresh Vegetable Pasty
Potato, Cheese & Onion Pasty
Top Crust Steak & Kidney Pie
Top Crust Steak & Mushroom
    Pie
Top Crust Poachers Pie
Baked Mince Beef Roll
Beef & Onion Pie
Chicken & Onion Pie
Steak & Kidney Pie

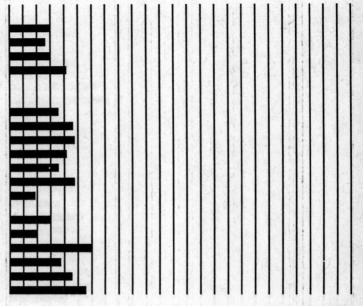

♦ = negligible

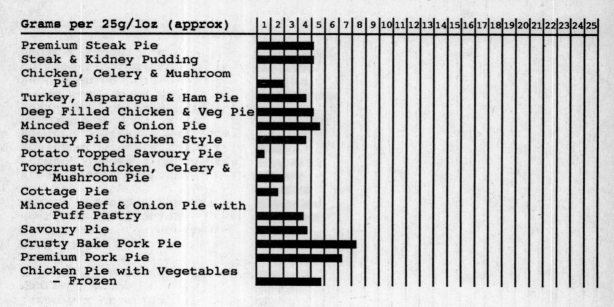

Grams per 25g/1oz (approx)	1	2	3	4	5	6	7	8	9	10	11	12	13	14	15	16	17	18	19	20	21	22	23	24	25
Premium Steak Pie																									
Steak & Kidney Pudding																									
Chicken, Celery & Mushroom Pie																									
Turkey, Asparagus & Ham Pie																									
Deep Filled Chicken & Veg Pie																									
Minced Beef & Onion Pie																									
Savoury Pie Chicken Style																									
Potato Topped Savoury Pie																									
Topcrust Chicken, Celery & Mushroom Pie																									
Cottage Pie																									
Minced Beef & Onion Pie with Puff Pastry																									
Savoury Pie																									
Crusty Bake Pork Pie																									
Premium Pork Pie																									
Chicken Pie with Vegetables – Frozen																									

291

Smoked Ham & Peppers Quiche
    - Frozen

TESCO

Frozen
Buffet Pork Pies
Beef in Ale Top Crust Pie
Beefsteak Pie – Family
Chicken & Asparagus Pie
Chicken & Vegetable Pie
Chicken Pie – Family
Chicken, Wine & Cream Top
    Crust Pie
Ham Leek & Cheese Pie
King Size Sausage Rolls
Minced Beef & Onion Pie
Minced Beef & Vegetable Pie
Pork, Apple & Cider Top
    Crust Pie
Steak & Kidney Pie – Family

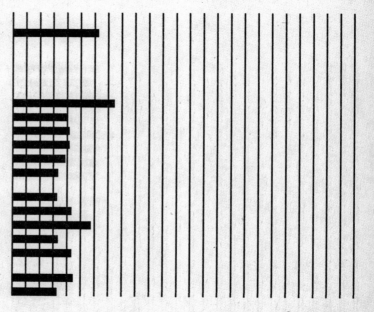

♦ = negligible

Grams per 25g/1oz (approx)	Grams
Steak & Mushroom Pie – Family	4
Steak Pie	4
Vegetable Pie	4
Chilled	
Chicken & Ham Pie with Sweetcorn Relish	4
Chicken, Sage & Onion Pie	6
Crispy Bake Buffet Pork Pies	7
Crispy Bake Chicken and Ham Buffet Pies	6
Crispy Bake Mini Pork Pies	6
Crispy Bake Pork Pie	6
Lattice Pork Pie	7
Melton Mowbray Pork Pie	6
Melton Mowbray Buffet Pork Pies	7
Mini Sausage Rolls	6
Pork & Egg Pie	6

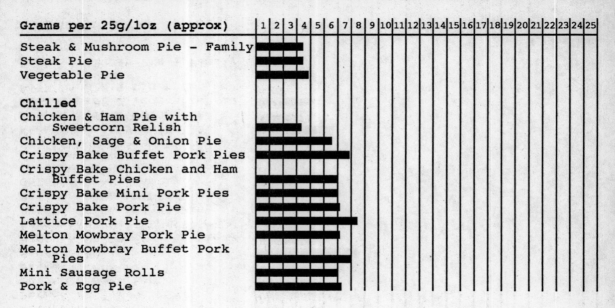

293

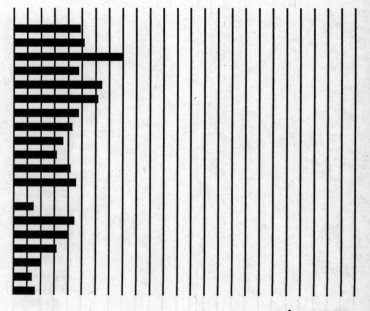

Pork & Gammon Pie with Pineapple
Pork & Onion Plait
Pork & Paté Pie
Potato & Meat Pie
Premium Pork Pie
Sausage Rolls
Bacon & Onion Roll
Baked Bean & Bacon Snacks
Beef & Onion Pasty
Beef & Onion Quorn Pie
Chicken & Leek Pie
Chicken & Mushroom Pie
Chicken & Mushroom Potato Topped Pie
Chicken & Vegetable Pie
Chunky Vegetable Roll
Cornish Pasty
Cottage Pie
Crofters Pie
Cumberland Pie

294

♦ = negligible

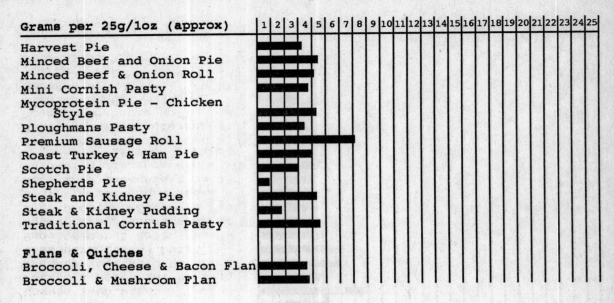

Grams per 25g/1oz (approx)	1	2	3	4	5	6	7	8	9	10	11	12	13	14	15	16	17	18	19	20	21	22	23	24	25
Harvest Pie																									
Minced Beef and Onion Pie																									
Minced Beef & Onion Roll																									
Mini Cornish Pasty																									
Mycoprotein Pie – Chicken Style																									
Ploughmans Pasty																									
Premium Sausage Roll																									
Roast Turkey & Ham Pie																									
Scotch Pie																									
Shepherds Pie																									
Steak and Kidney Pie																									
Steak & Kidney Pudding																									
Traditional Cornish Pasty																									

Flans & Quiches

| Broccoli, Cheese & Bacon Flan | | | | | | | | | | | | | | | | | | | | | | | | | |
| Broccoli & Mushroom Flan | | | | | | | | | | | | | | | | | | | | | | | | | |

Cheese & Broccoli Quiche Wedge	
Cheese & Onion Flan	
Cheese & Onion Mini Quiche	
Cheese & Onion Quiche Wedge	
Country Vegetable Quiche	
Deep Dish Quiche Lorraine	
Egg, Cheese & Bacon Flan	
Egg, Cheese & Bacon Quiche	
Egg, Cheese & Broccoli Flan	
Egg, Cheese & Onion Flan	
Egg, Ham, Cheese & Tomato Quiche	
Fishermans Flan	
Ham & Tomato Quiche Wedge	
Ham, Tomato & Cheese Mini Quiche	
Sausage, Bacon & Egg Quiche	
Spinach & Wholemeal Quiche	
Tuna & Tomato Quiche	
Tomato Egg & Cheese Flan	

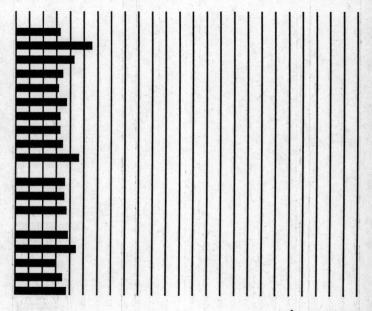

♦ = negligible

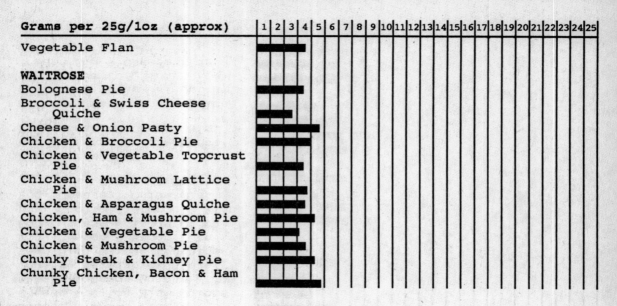

Grams per 25g/1oz (approx)	value
Vegetable Flan	4½
WAITROSE	
Bolognese Pie	4
Broccoli & Swiss Cheese Quiche	4
Cheese & Onion Pasty	5
Chicken & Broccoli Pie	4½
Chicken & Vegetable Topcrust Pie	4½
Chicken & Mushroom Lattice Pie	4½
Chicken & Asparagus Quiche	4½
Chicken, Ham & Mushroom Pie	4½
Chicken & Vegetable Pie	4
Chicken & Mushroom Pie	4½
Chunky Steak & Kidney Pie	4½
Chunky Chicken, Bacon & Ham Pie	5

Chunky Steak Pie
Cocktail Sausage Rolls
Cornish Pasty
Family Cottage Pie
Farmhouse Pork Pie
Gala Pork, Ham & Egg Pie
Ham & Cheese Mini Quiche
Ham & Cheese Quiche
Individual Pork Pie
Jamaican Patty
Lamb Samosa
Melton Mowbray Pork Pie
Minced Beef Pie
Mini Pork Pie
Oval Pork Pie
Pakora
Pan Italia
Pizza Pie
Pork & Egg Slices
Pork & Chicken Pie
Premium Cornish Pasty

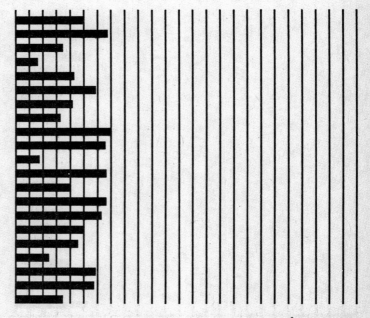

298

♦ = negligible

Grams per 25g/1oz (approx)	1	2	3	4	5	6	7	8	9	10	11	12	13	14	15	16	17	18	19	20	21	22	23	24	25
Savoury Minced Beef Pasty	████████████																								
Spring Roll	██																								
Steak & Kidney Pie	██████																								
Steak & Mushroom Pie	████████																								
Steak, Mushroom & Red Wine Pie	████																								
Steak & Kidney Pudding	██████																								
Steak & Mushroom Pie	███████																								
Turkey & Chestnut Pie	████████																								
Vegetable Samosa	███████																								
Vegetable Burrito	█																								

PIZZAS

ICELAND

	1	2	3	4	5	6	7	8	9	10	11	12	13	14	15	16	17	18	19	20	21	22	23	24	25
Barbecue Beef	████																								
Cheese & Tomato	████																								
Deep Chilli Beef	████																								
Garlic Pizza Bread	████████																								

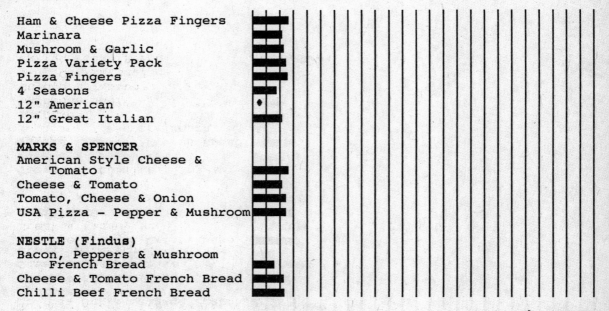

Ham & Cheese Pizza Fingers
Marinara
Mushroom & Garlic
Pizza Variety Pack
Pizza Fingers
4 Seasons
12" American
12" Great Italian

MARKS & SPENCER
American Style Cheese &
   Tomato
Cheese & Tomato
Tomato, Cheese & Onion
USA Pizza – Pepper & Mushroom

NESTLE (Findus)
Bacon, Peppers & Mushroom
   French Bread
Cheese & Tomato French Bread
Chilli Beef French Bread

◆ = negligible

Grams per 25g/1oz (approx)	1	2	3	4	5	6	7	8	9	10	11	12	13	14	15	16	17	18	19	20	21	22	23	24	25
Italian Style Sausage French Bread	■																								
Pineapple & Ham French Bread	■																								
Sweetcorn, Pepper & Pineapple French Bread	■																								
Cheese & Tomato Crispy Base	■	■																							

SAINSBURYS

Frozen

	1	2	3	4	5	6	7	8	9	10	11	12	13	14	15	16	17	18	19	20	21	22	23	24	25
Cheese & Onion	■																								
Cheese & Tomato	■	■																							
Cheese & Tomato French Bread	■	■																							
Mushroom & Pepper French Bread	■	■																							
Pepperoni Sausage	■																								

Fresh
Cheese & Tomato
Cheese & Tomato & Mushroom

TESCO

Fresh
Cheese & Mushroom
Cheese & Tomato
Cheese & Tomato (Small)
Crispy Base with Bacon and
    Pepper
Crispy Base with Cheese and
    Tomato
Family Pizza with Vegetables
    & Spicy Sausage
Garlic & Herb Bread
Pan Bake with Tomato and
    Cheese
Pizza Bases
Pizza Al Mare

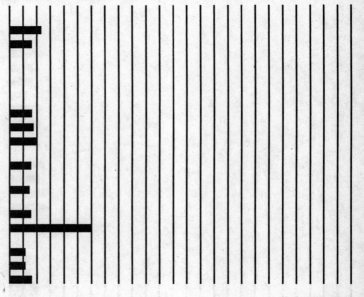

302

♦ = negligible

Grams per 25g/1oz (approx)	1	2	3	4	5	6	7	8	9	10	11	12	13	14	15	16	17	18	19	20	21	22	23	24	25
Pizza Italiana	██																								
Pizza Premier	██▌																								
Pizza Provencale	██▌																								
Pizza Snack with Mushroom	█▌																								
Frozen																									
Cheese & Tomato French Bread Pizza	███																								
Cheese & Onion Pizza	██▌																								
Cheese & Tomato Pizza	██																								
Ham & Mushroom Pizza	███																								
WAITROSE																									
Tomato & Cheese French Bread	██																								
Ham & Mushroom French Bread	█▌																								
Pizza Compagnola	██																								
Pizza Marinara	██																								
Pizza Pepperoni	██																								
Four Cheese	███																								

Luxury Pan Bake
Pizza Bites
Cheese & Tomato Deep Pan
Vegetable & Spicy Sausage
Chilli Pan Bake Pizza
Cheese & Tomato Pan Bake
Tuna & Artichoke
Pizza Pie

POULTRY & POULTRY DISHES –
GENERAL
Chicken, Boiled:
Meat only
Light Meat
Dark Meat
Chicken, Roast:
Meat only
Meat and Skin
Light Meat
Dark Meat

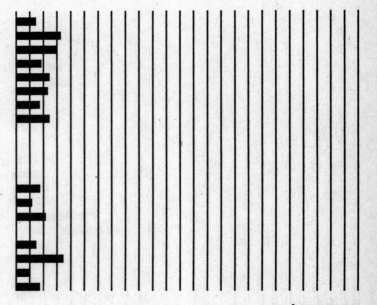

304

♦ = negligible

Grams per 25g/1oz (approx)	1	2	3	4	5	6	7	8	9	10	11	12	13	14	15	16	17	18	19	20	21	22	23	24	25

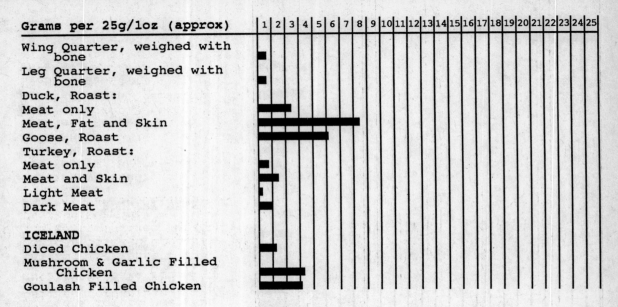

Wing Quarter, weighed with bone

Leg Quarter, weighed with bone

Duck, Roast:

Meat only

Meat, Fat and Skin

Goose, Roast

Turkey, Roast:

Meat only

Meat and Skin

Light Meat

Dark Meat

ICELAND

Diced Chicken

Mushroom & Garlic Filled Chicken

Goulash Filled Chicken

Garlic & Herb Chicken
    Drumsticks
Chicken Kiev
Chicken Cordon Bleu
Chicken Breast with Garlic
    Cheese
Chicken Italienne
Mexican Chicken Breasts
Italienne Chicken Breasts
Chicken Quarters
Southern Fried Chicken
    Portion
Chicken Thighs
Southern Fried Chicken
    Drumsticks
Chicken Breasts
Chicken Drumsticks
Roast Chicken Portions
Roast Chicken Drumsticks
Chicken Fingers
Chicken Nibbles

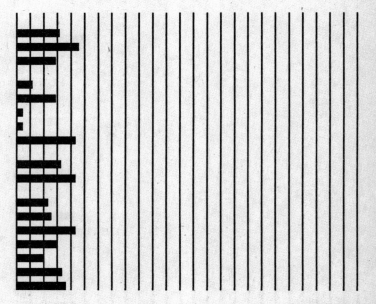

♦ = negligible

Grams per 25g/1oz (approx)

Item	1	2	3	4	5	6	7	8	9	10	11	12	13	14	15	16	17	18	19	20	21	22	23	24	25
Part Boned Chicken Breasts					█																				
Chicken Breast Fillets	█																								
Trimmed Chicken Legs				█																					
Chicken Breasts with Korma Filling	█																								
Chicken Breasts with Lemon & Peppers					█																				
Chicken Breasteaks					█																				
Chicken Tikka				█																					
Chinese Style Chicken Wings			█																						
Chicken Goujons					█																				
Teriyaki Chicken Breasts	█																								
Mustard & Honey Chicken Breasts		█																							
Hot & Spicy Wings				█																					
Premium Fresh Style British Chicken	█																								
Chinese Style Chicken Breasts	█																								
Tikka Style Chicken Breasts	█																								

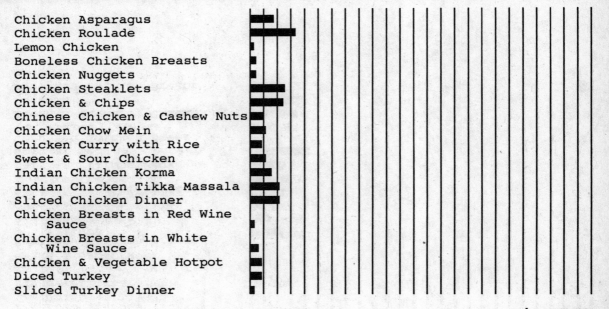

Chicken Asparagus
Chicken Roulade
Lemon Chicken
Boneless Chicken Breasts
Chicken Nuggets
Chicken Steaklets
Chicken & Chips
Chinese Chicken & Cashew Nuts
Chicken Chow Mein
Chicken Curry with Rice
Sweet & Sour Chicken
Indian Chicken Korma
Indian Chicken Tikka Massala
Sliced Chicken Dinner
Chicken Breasts in Red Wine Sauce
Chicken Breasts in White Wine Sauce
Chicken & Vegetable Hotpot
Diced Turkey
Sliced Turkey Dinner

◆ = negligible

308

Grams per 25g/1oz (approx)	1	2	3	4	5	6	7	8	9	10	11	12	13	14	15	16	17	18	19	20	21	22	23	24	25
Traditional Roast Turkey Joint	■																								
Turkey Fillets	◆																								
MARKS & SPENCER																									
Boneless Chicken Breast Fillets			■																						
Boneless Thighs		■																							
Chicken Breast Fillets		■																							
Chicken Breast Fillets – Free Range		■																							
Chicken Fillets Pack			■																						
Chicken Legs				■																					
Corn Fed Chicken Breast Fillet		■																							
Fresh Oven Ready Chicken			■																						
Poussin			■																						
Boneless Chicken Breast		■																							

Breaded Chicken Thighs & Drums	
Chicken Bites	
Chicken Breast Fillets in Breadcrumbs	
Chicken Breast Fillets - Breaded	
Chicken Goujons	
Chicken Liver Paté	
Chicken Medallions	
Chilli Chicken - Cooked	
Chinese Kebab with Sweet & Sour Sauce	
Chinese Style Chicken	
Honey & Mustard Breast Fillets	
Roast Assortment Pack	
Roast Breast Fillets	
Roast Chicken Strips	
Roast Turkey Sliced	

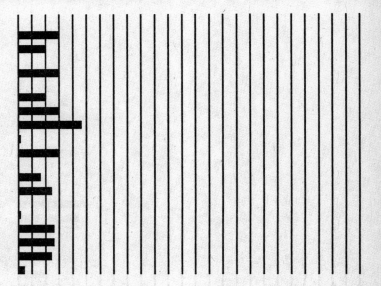

310

♦ = negligible

Grams per 25g/1oz (approx)	1	2	3	4	5	6	7	8	9	10	11	12	13	14	15	16	17	18	19	20	21	22	23	24	25

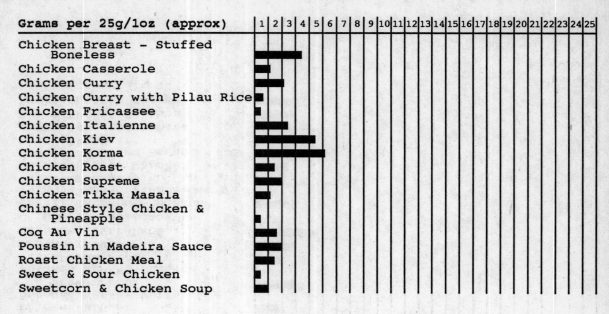

Chicken Breast - Stuffed Boneless				
Chicken Casserole	
Chicken Curry		
Chicken Curry with Pilau Rice	
Chicken Fricassee	
Chicken Italienne		
Chicken Kiev				
Chicken Korma					
Chicken Roast	
Chicken Supreme	
Chicken Tikka Masala	
Chinese Style Chicken & Pineapple	
Coq Au Vin		
Poussin in Madeira Sauce		
Roast Chicken Meal		
Sweet & Sour Chicken	
Sweetcorn & Chicken Soup	

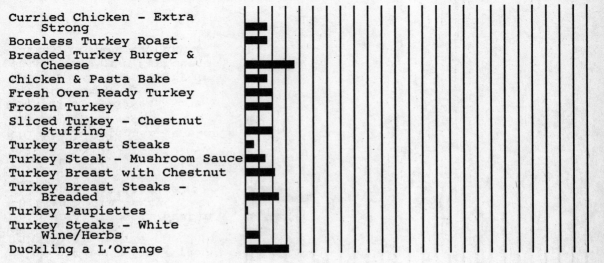

Curried Chicken - Extra Strong	
Boneless Turkey Roast	
Breaded Turkey Burger & Cheese	
Chicken & Pasta Bake	
Fresh Oven Ready Turkey	
Frozen Turkey	
Sliced Turkey - Chestnut Stuffing	
Turkey Breast Steaks	
Turkey Steak - Mushroom Sauce	
Turkey Breast with Chestnut	
Turkey Breast Steaks - Breaded	
Turkey Paupiettes	
Turkey Steaks - White Wine/Herbs	
Duckling a L'Orange	

♦ = negligible

Grams per 25g/1oz (approx)	1	2	3	4	5	6	7	8	9	10	11	12	13	14	15	16	17	18	19	20	21	22	23	24	25
NESTLE (Crosse & Blackwell)																									
Chicken Curry with Separate Rice	█																								
Findus																									
Cashew Chicken	██																								
Chicken & Broccoli Gratin	███																								
Chicken Korma Curry	██																								
Chicken & Tagliatelle	███																								
Lean Cuisine																									
Chicken a L'Orange	█																								
Chicken & Oriental Vegetable	█																								
Chicken Cacciatore	█																								
Chicken Primavera	█																								
Glazed Chicken	█																								
Kashmiri Chicken Curry	█																								
Chicken & Prawn Cantonese	█																								
Turkey in Mushroom Sauce	█																								

SAINSBURYS

Chicken Breasts – Roast or Grill

Chicken Drumsticks – Roast or Grill

Chicken Leg Portions – Oven Baked

Chicken Quarters – Roast or Grill

Chicken Thighs – Oven Baked

Chicken Boneless Thighs – Oven Baked

Chicken Livers – Fried in Butter

Chargrill Flavoured Chicken Breast – Baked

Chargrill Flavoured Chicken Leg – Baked

Premium Chickens

Roasting Chickens

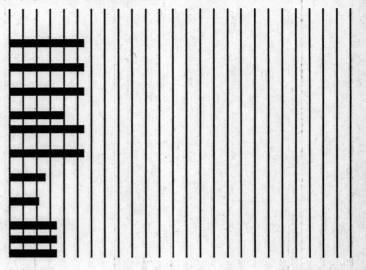

314

◆ = negligible

Grams per 25g/1oz (approx)	1	2	3	4	5	6	7	8	9	10	11	12	13	14	15	16	17	18	19	20	21	22	23	24	25
Chicken with Pork, Sage, Onion & Thyme Stuffing				▇																					
Chicken with Traditional Pork & Chestnut Stuffing			▇																						
Chicken Breast in Breadcrumbs - Baked		▇																							
Boneless Chicken in Breadcrumbs					▇																				
Chicken Breast in Wholewheat Breadcrumbs		▇																							
Breaded Chicken Nibbles - Baked				▇																					
Breaded Chicken Nuggets - Baked					▇																				
Chicken Goujons - Baked			▇																						
Chicken Breasts en Croute - Baked				▇																					
Quick Cook Chicken with Garlic & Parsley				▇																					

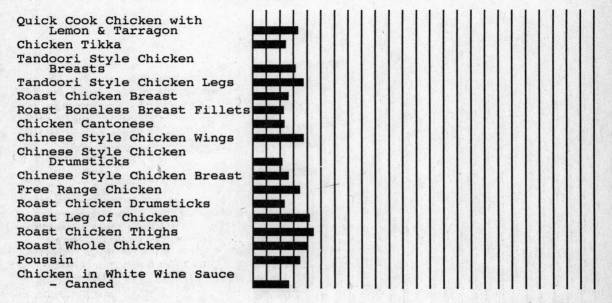

Quick Cook Chicken with
    Lemon & Tarragon
Chicken Tikka
Tandoori Style Chicken
    Breasts
Tandoori Style Chicken Legs
Roast Chicken Breast
Roast Boneless Breast Fillets
Chicken Cantonese
Chinese Style Chicken Wings
Chinese Style Chicken
    Drumsticks
Chinese Style Chicken Breast
Free Range Chicken
Roast Chicken Drumsticks
Roast Leg of Chicken
Roast Chicken Thighs
Roast Whole Chicken
Poussin
Chicken in White Wine Sauce
    - Canned

♦ = negligible

Grams per 25g/1oz (approx)	1	2	3	4	5	6	7	8	9	10	11	12	13	14	15	16	17	18	19	20	21	22	23	24	25
Chicken Breast – Canned	■																								
Chicken Kiev	■■■																								
Chicken Leek & Broccoli Bake	■■																								
Sweet & Sour Chicken	▪																								
Pineapple Chicken & Barbecue Beef	▪																								
Chicken Tikka Masala	■■																								
Chicken Steaks Italian Style	■■■																								
Chicken Cacciatore	■■																								
Chicken Lasagne – Frozen	■																								
Chicken Kiev	■■■■																								
Chicken with Oriental Vegetables – Stir Fry	▪																								
Diced Boneless Turkey	▪																								
Oven Ready Turkey	■■																								
Turkey Livers – Fried	■■■																								
Turkey Breast Fillet – Baked	▪																								
Turkey Breast Slices	▪																								
Duckling	■■■■■■																								

Duckling a L'Orange

TESCO

Chicken
Breast Fillet, Skinless
Breast, Meat and Skin
Breast, Meat Only
Casserole Hen, Meat Only
Cornfed, Meat and Skin
Cornfed, Meat Only
Drumsticks, Meat and Skin
Drumsticks, Meat Only
Poussin, Meat Only
Quarters, Meat and Skin
Quarters, Meat Only
Whole Chicken, Meat and Skin
Whole Chicken, Meat Only
Wings, Meat and Skin
Wings, Meat Only
Boneless Stuffed Chicken

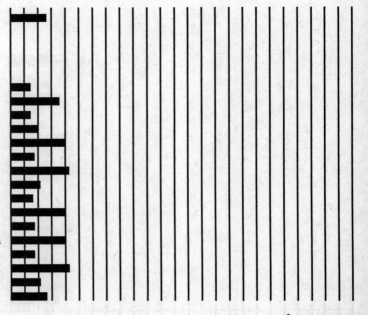

♦ = negligible

Grams per 25g/1oz (approx)

Scale columns: 1 2 3 4 5 6 7 8 9 10 11 12 13 14 15 16 17 18 19 20 21 22 23 24 25

Food	Grams per 25g/1oz (approx)
Cooked Whole Chicken	~4
Whole Roast Chicken	~4.5
Roast Chicken Breasts	~3.5
Roast Chicken Drumsticks	~3
Roast Chicken Portion	~4.5
Roast Chicken Thighs	~5
Chicken – Products	
American Style Chicken Portion – Breaded	~4
American Style Chicken Drumsticks – Breaded	~4
Breaded Chicken Steaks	~4
Chargrill Chicken Breast	~3
Chargrill Chicken Drumstick	~3
Chargrill Whole Chicken	~4.5
Chicken Cordon Bleu – Breaded	~3
Chicken En Croute with Mushroom & Cheese	~4.5

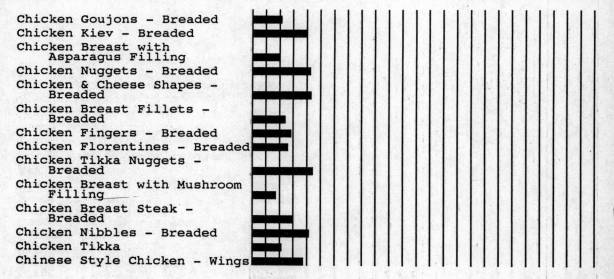

Chicken Goujons - Breaded
Chicken Kiev - Breaded
Chicken Breast with
    Asparagus Filling
Chicken Nuggets - Breaded
Chicken & Cheese Shapes -
    Breaded
Chicken Breast Fillets -
    Breaded
Chicken Fingers - Breaded
Chicken Florentines - Breaded
Chicken Tikka Nuggets -
    Breaded
Chicken Breast with Mushroom
    Filling
Chicken Breast Steak -
    Breaded
Chicken Nibbles - Breaded
Chicken Tikka
Chinese Style Chicken - Wings

320

♦ = negligible

Grams per 25g/1oz (approx)	1	2	3	4	5	6	7	8	9	10	11	12	13	14	15	16	17	18	19	20	21	22	23	24	25
Chinese Style Chicken – Breast	███																								
Curried Chicken – Portion	███																								
Garlic Basted Chicken	███																								
Garlic Chicken	████																								
Korma Bites	███																								
Lemon, Parsley & Thyme Stuffed Chicken	███																								
Lemon Chicken	████																								
Masala Chicken Drumsticks	███																								
Mexican Bites	███																								
Pork, Sage & Onion Stuffed Chicken	███																								
Premium Chicken Nuggets – Breaded	███																								
Ready Basted Chicken	███																								
Reformed Chicken Cordon Bleu – Breaded	██																								

321

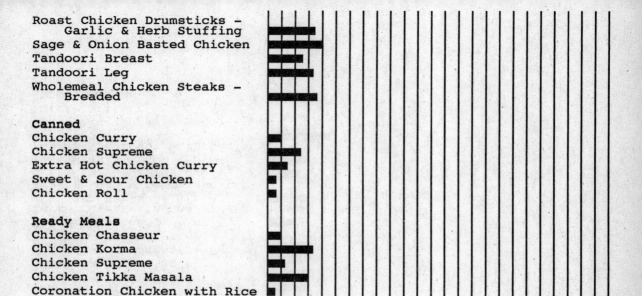

Roast Chicken Drumsticks –
Garlic & Herb Stuffing
Sage & Onion Basted Chicken
Tandoori Breast
Tandoori Leg
Wholemeal Chicken Steaks –
Breaded

Canned
Chicken Curry
Chicken Supreme
Extra Hot Chicken Curry
Sweet & Sour Chicken
Chicken Roll

Ready Meals
Chicken Chasseur
Chicken Korma
Chicken Supreme
Chicken Tikka Masala
Coronation Chicken with Rice

322

ϕ = negligible

Grams per 25g/1oz (approx)	1	2	3	4	5	6	7	8	9	10	11	12	13	14	15	16	17	18	19	20	21	22	23	24	25

Turkey

Item	Grams per 25g/1oz (approx)
Boneless Joint	2
Boneless Stuffed Joint	2
Boneless Turkey Roast	2.5
Cured Turkey Breast – Canned	1
Thighs, Meat Only	2
Thighs, Meat and Skin	2.5
Turkey Steaks in Red Wine & Herb Marinade	4.5
Turkey Loaf with Cheese & Potato Topping	2.5
Turkey Wellington	3
Turkey En Croute with Garlic & Cheese Sauce	5
Turkey Escalopes	1
Turkey Stir Fry	1
Turkey Steaks	1
Turkey Mince	1

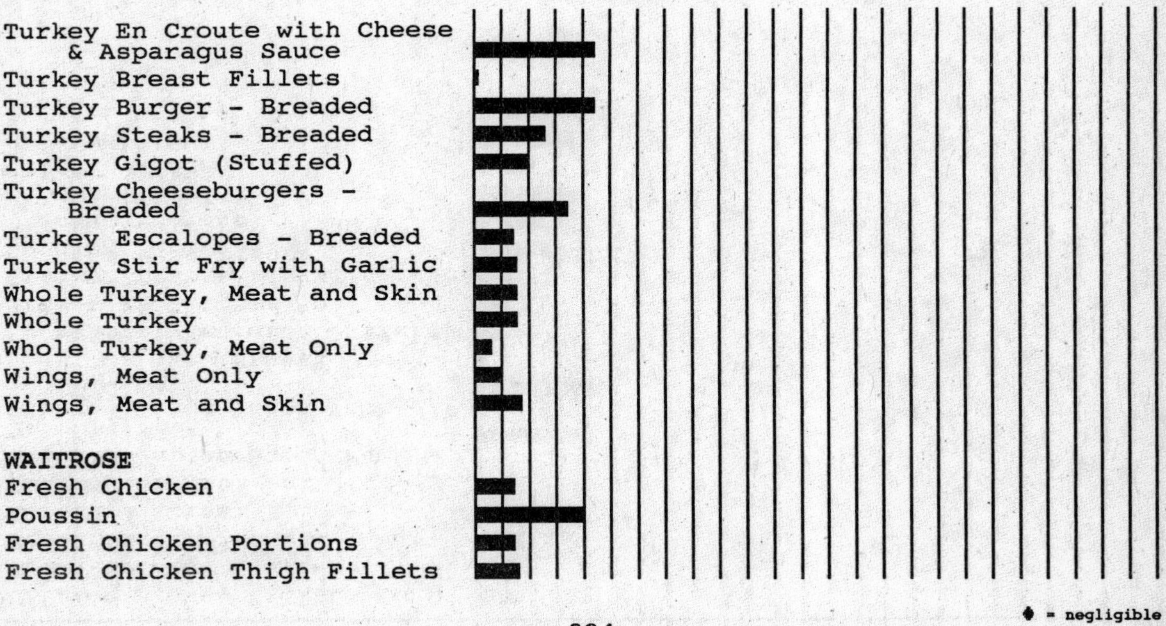

Turkey En Croute with Cheese & Asparagus Sauce

Turkey Breast Fillets

Turkey Burger - Breaded

Turkey Steaks - Breaded

Turkey Gigot (Stuffed)

Turkey Cheeseburgers - Breaded

Turkey Escalopes - Breaded

Turkey Stir Fry with Garlic

Whole Turkey, Meat and Skin

Whole Turkey

Whole Turkey, Meat Only

Wings, Meat Only

Wings, Meat and Skin

WAITROSE

Fresh Chicken

Poussin

Fresh Chicken Portions

Fresh Chicken Thigh Fillets

♦ = negligible

Grams per 25g/1oz (approx)

Food	Grams per 25g/1oz (approx)
Chicken Breast Fillet	2
Fresh Chicken Quarters	2
Fresh Chicken Legs	2
Frozen Chicken	4
Chicken Livers	2
Chicken Thighs Pouch Pack – Frozen	5
Chicken Wings Pouch Pack – Frozen	5
Roast Chicken Breast	1
Cooked Chicken with Stuffing	1
Breast of Chicken Roll	2
Chicken Creole	2
Chicken Cordon Bleu	3
Chicken Goujons	3
Chicken Kiev	5
Chicken Madras	2
Chicken Nibbles	4
Chicken Olives	4

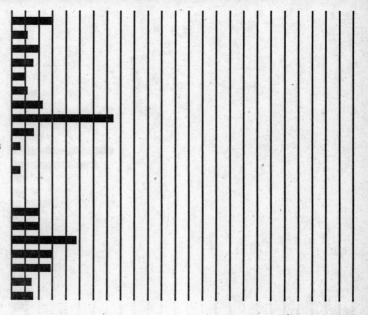

Chicken Paté
Chicken Roll
Chicken Romane
Chicken Samosa
Chicken Sate Sticks
Chicken Tandoori
Chicken Tikka
Coronation Chicken
Hawaiian Chicken
Indian Style Chicken Nibbles
Smoky Barbecue Chicken
    Nibbles

Ready Meals
Tandoori Chicken Masala
Mild Chicken Curry
Chicken Korma Curry
Chicken Spring Roll
Chicken with Almonds
Chicken Casserole
Chicken Moghlai

♦ = negligible

326

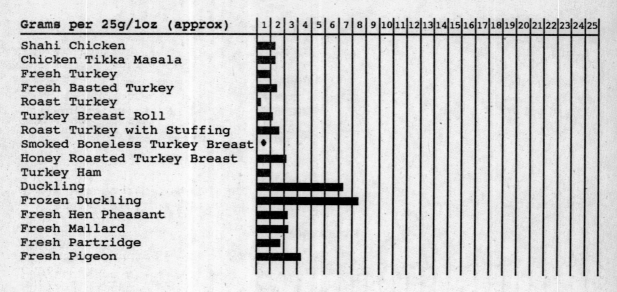

Grams per 25g/1oz (approx)

	1	2	3	4	5	6	7	8	9	10	11	12	13	14	15	16	17	18	19	20	21	22	23	24	25
Shahi Chicken																									
Chicken Tikka Masala																									
Fresh Turkey																									
Fresh Basted Turkey																									
Roast Turkey																									
Turkey Breast Roll																									
Roast Turkey with Stuffing																									
Smoked Boneless Turkey Breast																									
Honey Roasted Turkey Breast																									
Turkey Ham																									
Duckling																									
Frozen Duckling																									
Fresh Hen Pheasant																									
Fresh Mallard																									
Fresh Partridge																									
Fresh Pigeon																									

PUDDINGS & DESSERTS - GENERAL

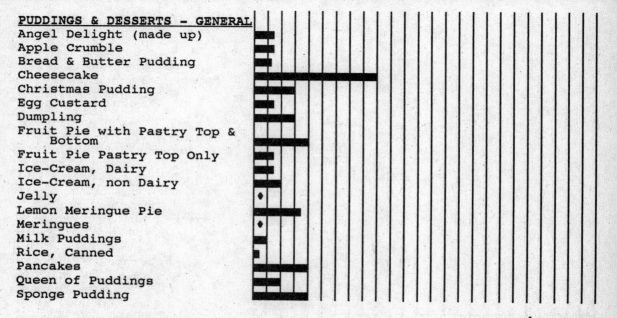

Angel Delight (made up)
Apple Crumble
Bread & Butter Pudding
Cheesecake
Christmas Pudding
Egg Custard
Dumpling
Fruit Pie with Pastry Top & Bottom
Fruit Pie Pastry Top Only
Ice-Cream, Dairy
Ice-Cream, non Dairy
Jelly
Lemon Meringue Pie
Meringues
Milk Puddings
Rice, Canned
Pancakes
Queen of Puddings
Sponge Pudding

♦ = negligible

Grams per 25g/1oz (approx)	1 2 3 4 5 6 7 8 9 10 11 12 13 14 15 16 17 18 19 20 21 22 23 24 25
Suet Pudding	▉▉▉▉▉
Treacle Tart	▉▉▉▉
Trifle	▉
Yorkshire Pudding	▉▉▉
CO-OP	
Chocolate Sponge Pudding	▉▉▉
Christmas Pudding	▉▉
Lemon Sponge Pudding	▉▉▉
Low Fat Rice Pudding	▏
Macaroni Pudding	▏
Mixed Fruit Sponge Pudding	▉▉▉
Raspberry Sponge Pudding	▉▉▉
Rice Pudding	▏
Sago Pudding	
Semolina Pudding	▏
Strawberry Sponge Pudding	▉▉▉
Syrup Sponge Pudding	▉▉
Tapioca Pudding	▏

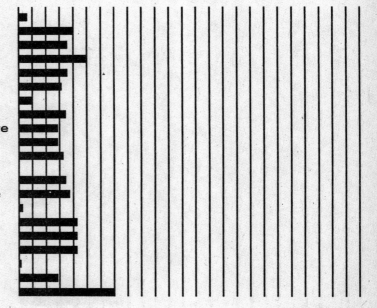

Traditional Rice Pudding
Blackcurrant Cheesecake
Morello Cherry Cheesecake
Black Forest Gateau
Strawberry Gateau
Deep Dish Apple Pie
Chunky Apple Crumble
Family Apple Pie
Chocolate Dairy Cream Sponge
Dairy Cream Sponge
Dairy Cream & Apple Cake
Morello Cherry Dairy Cream
    Cake
Strawberry Dairy Cream Cake
Batter Mix
Crumble Mix
Fairy Cake Mix
Luxury Sponge Mix
Rock Cake Base Mix
Scone Mix
Short Pastry Mix

◆ = negligible

330

Grams per 25g/1oz (approx)	1	2	3	4	5	6	7	8	9	10	11	12	13	14	15	16	17	18	19	20	21	22	23	24	25
Suet Dumpling Mix	██	██	██	██	██	██	██	██																	
Butterscotch Dessert Whip	◆																								
Raspberry Dessert Whip	◆																								
Strawberry Dessert Whip	◆																								
Banana Supreme Delight	██	██																							
Chocolate Supreme Delight	██	██																							
Raspberry Supreme Delight	██	██																							
Strawberry Supreme Delight	██	██																							
Banana Sugar Free Supreme Delight	██	██	██																						
Chocolate Sugar Free Supreme Delight	██	██	██																						
Lemon Sugar Free Supreme Delight	██	██	██																						
Orange Sugar Free Supreme Delight	██	██	██																						
Strawberry Sugar Free Supreme Delight	██	██	██																						

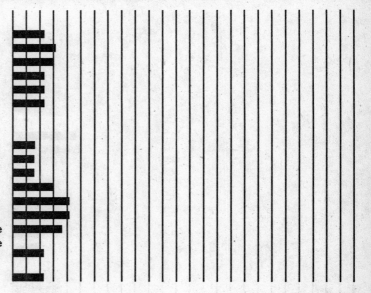

HEINZ
Apple & Blackberry Sponge
Chocolate Sponge
Mixed Fruit Sponge
Raspberry Jam Sponge
Strawberry Jam Sponge
Treacle Sponge

ICELAND
Banana Mousse
Chocolate Mousse
Strawberry Mousse
Strawberry Surprises
Fruits of Forest Torte
Raspberry & Chocolate Torte
Raspberry & Almond Dacquoise
Mint Flavour Choc Ripple Ice
    Cream Roll
Orange Flavoured Choc Ice
    Cream Roll

♦ = negligible

332

Grams per 25g/1oz (approx)   1 2 3 4 5 6 7 8 9 10 11 12 13 14 15 16 17 18 19 20 21 22 23 24 25

MARKS & SPENCER

Item	Grams per 25g/1oz (approx)
Apricot and Peach Pie	4
Banana Fool	2
Banana in Custard	1
Blackberry and Apple Fool	2
Blackcurrant Fruit Fool	2
Caramel Delight Dessert	2
Charlotte Russe	4
Chocolate Dairy Mousse	
Chocolate Delight Dessert	2
Chocolate Dessert	1
Chocolate Fudge Brownies	6
Chocolate Layer Cake	5
Chocolate Ripple	1
Chocolate Soufflé	2
Creme Caramel	2
Fresh Cream Banana Trifle	3
Fresh Fruit Salad	1

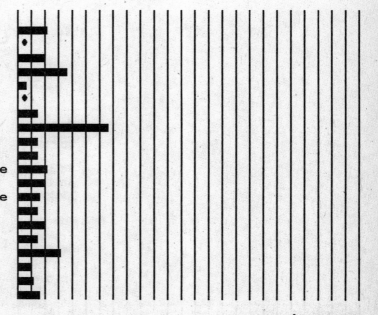

Gooseberry and Greengage Caprice	
Gooseberry Compote	◆
Gooseberry Fruit Fool	
Grape & Ginger Syllabub	
Honeydew Lemon Delight	
Mandarin in Orange Jelly	◆
Peach & Mango Delight	
Pot au Chocolate	
Raspberry Royale Dessert	
Raspberry Ring Dessert	
Rhubarb & Strawberry Caprice	
Rhubarb Fruit Fool	
Rice Dessert & Apricot Puree	
Rum Babas	
Sherry Trifle	
Strawberry & Guava Delight	
Strawberry Cream Gateau	
Strawberry Dairy Mousse	
Strawberry Delight Dessert	
Strawberry Fruit Fool	

◆ = negligible

334

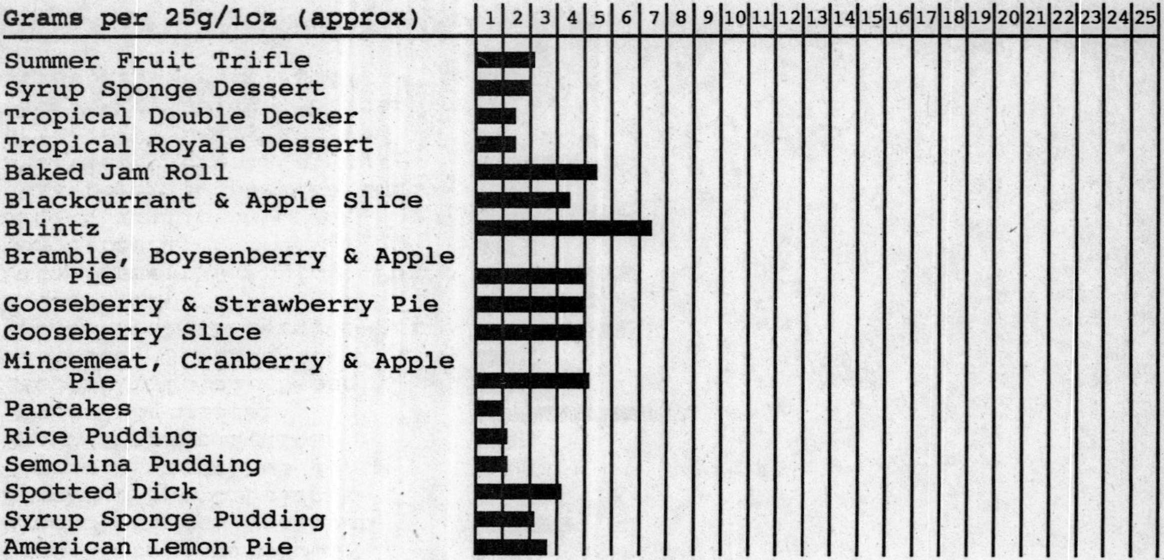

Grams per 25g/1oz (approx)   1 2 3 4 5 6 7 8 9 10 11 12 13 14 15 16 17 18 19 20 21 22 23 24 25

- Summer Fruit Trifle
- Syrup Sponge Dessert
- Tropical Double Decker
- Tropical Royale Dessert
- Baked Jam Roll
- Blackcurrant & Apple Slice
- Blintz
- Bramble, Boysenberry & Apple Pie
- Gooseberry & Strawberry Pie
- Gooseberry Slice
- Mincemeat, Cranberry & Apple Pie
- Pancakes
- Rice Pudding
- Semolina Pudding
- Spotted Dick
- Syrup Sponge Pudding
- American Lemon Pie

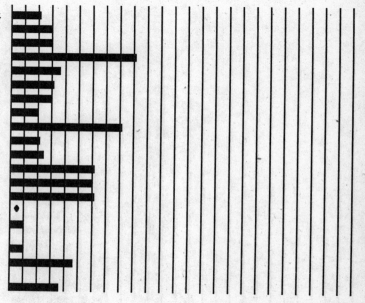

American Style Apple Dessert
American Style Danish
Apricot Cheesecake
Black Forest Gateau
Blackcurrant & Apple Pie
Blackcurrant Cheesecake
Cherry Cheesecake
Cherry Meringue Pie
Choux Ring Dessert
Deep Filled Apple Pie
Duchesse Dessert
Frozen Cream Doughnuts
Fudge Flan
Lemon Cream Flan
Lemon Torte
Lite Blackcurrant Cheesecake
Lite Tropical Fruit
  Cheesecake
Pecan Danish Pastry
Raspberry & Redcurrant
  Cheesecake

336

♦ = negligible

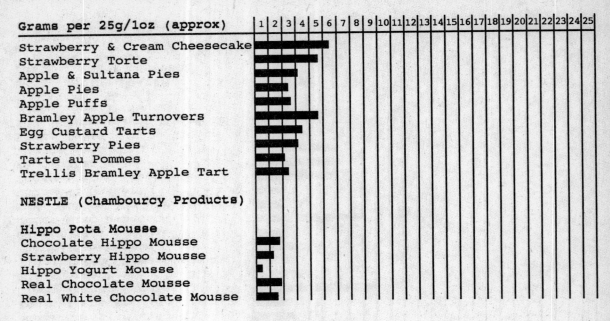

Grams per 25g/1oz (approx)	1	2	3	4	5	6	7	8	9	10	11	12	13	14	15	16	17	18	19	20	21	22	23	24	25
Strawberry & Cream Cheesecake																									
Strawberry Torte																									
Apple & Sultana Pies																									
Apple Pies																									
Apple Puffs																									
Bramley Apple Turnovers																									
Egg Custard Tarts																									
Strawberry Pies																									
Tarte au Pommes																									
Trellis Bramley Apple Tart																									

NESTLE (Chambourcy Products)

Hippo Pota Mousse
Chocolate Hippo Mousse
Strawberry Hippo Mousse
Hippo Yogurt Mousse
Real Chocolate Mousse
Real White Chocolate Mousse

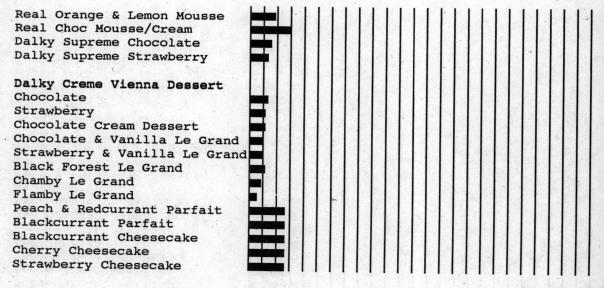

Real Orange & Lemon Mousse
Real Choc Mousse/Cream
Dalky Supreme Chocolate
Dalky Supreme Strawberry

Dalky Creme Vienna Dessert
Chocolate
Strawberry
Chocolate Cream Dessert
Chocolate & Vanilla Le Grand
Strawberry & Vanilla Le Grand
Black Forest Le Grand
Chamby Le Grand
Flamby Le Grand
Peach & Redcurrant Parfait
Blackcurrant Parfait
Blackcurrant Cheesecake
Cherry Cheesecake
Strawberry Cheesecake

338

♦ = negligible

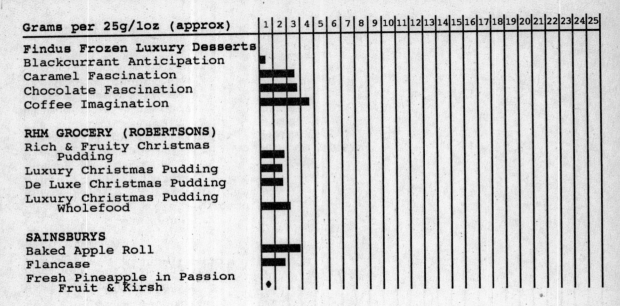

Grams per 25g/1oz (approx)	1	2	3	4	5	6	7	8	9	10	11	12	13	14	15	16	17	18	19	20	21	22	23	24	25

Findus Frozen Luxury Desserts
Blackcurrant Anticipation
Caramel Fascination
Chocolate Fascination
Coffee Imagination

RHM GROCERY (ROBERTSONS)
Rich & Fruity Christmas Pudding
Luxury Christmas Pudding
De Luxe Christmas Pudding
Luxury Christmas Pudding Wholefood

SAINSBURYS
Baked Apple Roll
Flancase
Fresh Pineapple in Passion Fruit & Kirsh

Golden Bake Flan Case
Gooseberry Fool
Jam Sponge
Meringue Pavlova
Meringue Pavlova and Crown
Meringue Nests
Rhubarb Fool
Shortcrust Pastry Case
Sweet Pastry Case
Trifle Sponges
Brambly Apple Pie – Frozen
Double Chocolate Gateau – Frozen
Nut Meringue Gateau – Frozen
Shortcrust Pastry – Frozen

ST IVEL
Devonshire Cheesecake – Blackcurrant
Devonshire Cheesecake – Lemon & Sultana

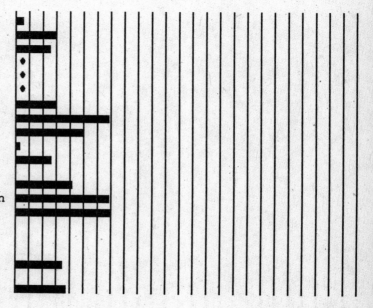

340

♦ = negligible

Grams per 25g/1oz (approx)	1	2	3	4	5	6	7	8	9	10	11	12	13	14	15	16	17	18	19	20	21	22	23	24	25
Devonshire Cheesecake - Strawberry	■	■	■																						
Fruit Cocktail Trifle	■																								
Mandarin Trifle	■																								
Peach Trifle	■	■																							
Raspberry Trifle	■	■																							
Strawberry Trifle	■																								
Black Forest Gateau	■	■	■																						
Strawberry Gateau	■	■	■	■																					
TESCO																									
Custard	■																								
Delight Mix (all flavours)	■	■																							
Dessert Toppings	■	■	■																						
Instant Custard	■																								
Jelly (all flavours)	♦																								
Sugar Free Delight - Butterscotch	■	■																							

Sugar Free Delight – Chocolate	
Sugar Free Delight – Strawberry	
Chilled	
Banana & Custard	
Black Cherry, Cream & Yogurt Double Dessert	
Blackcurrant Fool	
Caramel Dessert	
Caramel Supreme Dessert	
Childrens Strawberry Mousse	
Chocolate & Cherry Trifle	
Chocolate Nut Sundae	
Chocolate Sponge	
Chocolate Supreme Dessert	
Chocolate, Brandy & Orange Syllabub	
Custard Sauce	
Fruit Cocktail Trifle	

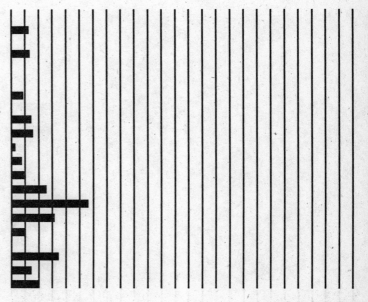

♦ = negligible

Grams per 25g/1oz (approx)	1	2	3	4	5	6	7	8	9	10	11	12	13	14	15	16	17	18	19	20	21	22	23	24	25
Gooseberry Fool																									
Honey, Cream & Yogurt Double Dessert																									
Luxury Chocolate Chip Mousse																									
Luxury Raspberry & Sherry Trifle																									
Luxury Strawberry Mousse																									
Peaches & Custard																									
Raspberry Sundae Turnout																									
Rhubarb Fool																									
Strawberries & Custard																									
Strawberry Flavoured Supreme Dessert																									
Strawberry Fool																									
Summer Fruit Dessert																									
Syrup Sponge																									

Frozen

Apple Crumble
Apple Strudel
Black Cherry Roulade
Black Forest Gateau
Blackcurrant & Apple Fruit Puffs
Blackcurrant Cheesecake
Bramley Apple Pie
Cherry Cheesecake
Cherry Pie
Chocolate & Mint Mousse
Chocolate Cheesecake
Chocolate Fudge Cake
Chocolate Meringue Gateau
Chocolate Orange Mousse
Choux Ring
Dairy Cream Sponge
Dutch Apple Pie
Economy Dairy Cream Sponge
Grand Marnier Gateau

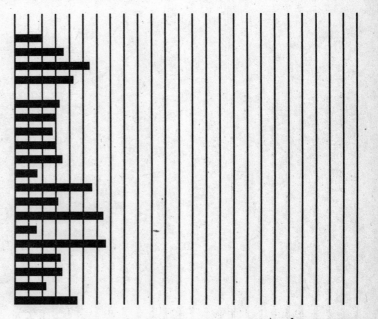

♦ = negligible

344

Grams per 25g/1oz (approx)	Grams
Lemon Cheesecake	5
Lemon Meringue Pie	2
Low Fat French Style Dessert – Chocolate	1
Low Fat French Style Dessert – Strawberry	1
Nut Meringue Gateau	7
Pineapple & Mandarin Gateau	3
Profiteroles	8
Raspberry Pavlova	4
Raspberry Ripple Mousse	2
Raspberry Shortcake	6
Strawberry & Cream Mousse	2
Strawberry Cheesecake	3
Strawberry Fruit Flan	2
Strawberry Gateau	3
Summer Fruit Crumble	2
Summer Fruit Flan	2

Toffee & Banana Flavour
    Mousse

WAITROSE
Jelly - (all flavours)
Banana Dessert
Butterscotch Dessert
Chocolate Orange Dessert
Mint Chocolate Dessert
Strawberry Dessert
Toffee Dessert
Vanilla Dessert
Chocolate Mousse
Raspberry Ripple Mousse
Strawberry/Cream Mousse
Toffee/Banana Mousse
Creamed Rice Pudding
Fruit Cocktail Trifle
Raspberry Trifle

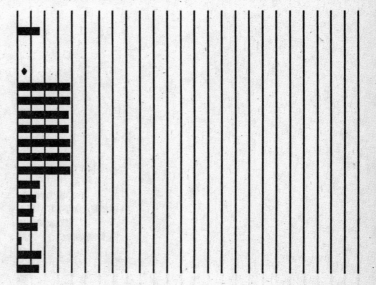

♦ = negligible

Grams per 25g/1oz (approx)	1	2	3	4	5	6	7	8	9	10	11	12	13	14	15	16	17	18	19	20	21	22	23	24	25

RICE & GRAINS - GENERAL
Cooked
Savoury - Dry Weight

MARKS & SPENCER
American Long Grain Rice
Basmati Rice
Natural Wholegrain Brown Rice

NESTLE (Crosse & Blackwell)

Rice & Things - Sachets
Curry
Italienne
Mushroom
Peppers
Vegetables

SAINSBURYS
Basmati – Cooked
Brown Rice – Boiled
Brown Rice – Canned
Easy Cook American Rice –
 Boiled
Easy Cook Italian Rice –
 Boiled
Flaked Rice
Ground Rice
Quick Cook Rice
Rice for Puddings
Semolina – Boiled
Canned Cream Rice
Traditional Canned Cream Rice
Chocolate Rice Pudding

Savoury Rices
Saffron Rice
Savoury Sweet & Sour Rice

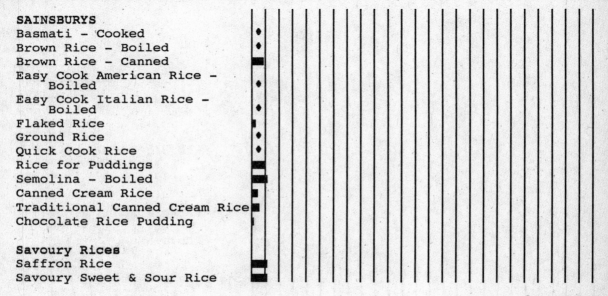

♦ = negligible

Grams per 25g/1oz (approx)	1	2	3	4	5	6	7	8	9	10	11	12	13	14	15	16	17	18	19	20	21	22	23	24	25
Savoury Brown with Peppers/Mushroom	▪																								
Savoury Golden Vegetable Rice	▪																								
Savoury Curry Rice	▪▪																								
Savoury Rice with Chicken/Sweetcorn	▪▪																								
Spiced Basmati Rice	▪																								
Vegetable Curry & Basmati Rice	▪																								
TESCO																									
American Easy Cook Rice	♦																								
American Long Grain Rice	♦																								
Basmati Rice	▪																								
Brown Rice	♦																								
Ground Rice	▪																								
Pearl Barley	♦																								
Pudding Rice	▪▪																								
Sago	▪▪																								

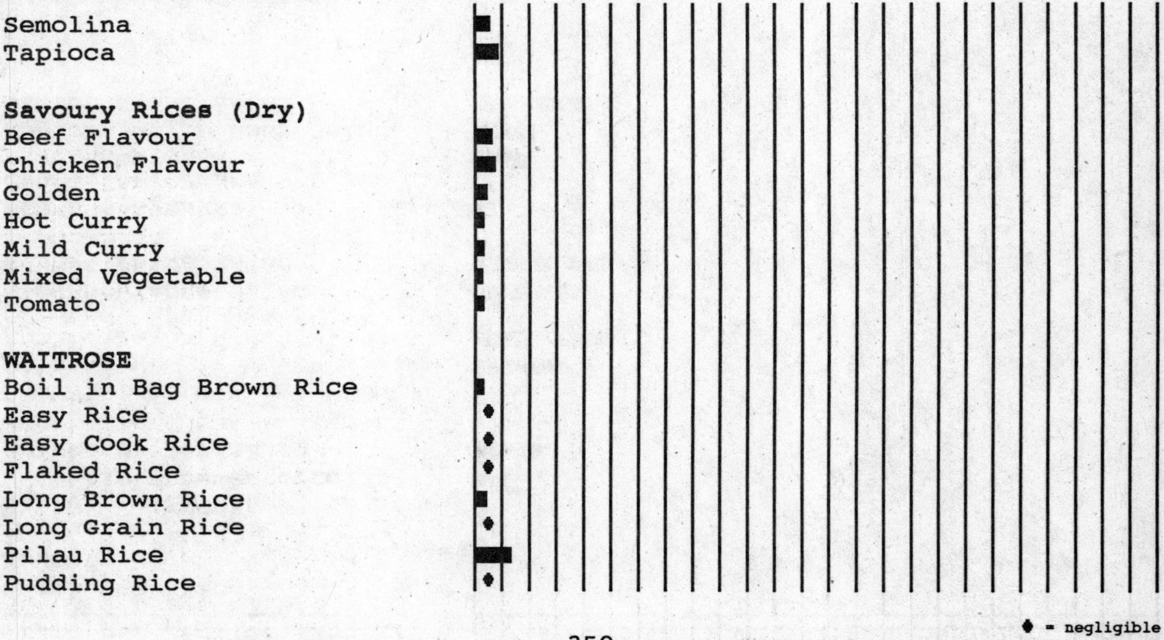

Semolina
Tapioca

Savoury Rices (Dry)
Beef Flavour
Chicken Flavour
Golden
Hot Curry
Mild Curry
Mixed Vegetable
Tomato

WAITROSE
Boil in Bag Brown Rice
Easy Rice
Easy Cook Rice
Flaked Rice
Long Brown Rice
Long Grain Rice
Pilau Rice
Pudding Rice

♦ = negligible

Grams per 25g/1oz (approx)	1	2	3	4	5	6	7	8	9	10	11	12	13	14	15	16	17	18	19	20	21	22	23	24	25
Quick Cook Rice	◆																								
Risotto Rice	◆																								

SALADS – GENERAL

Coleslaw, Low Calorie	■																								
Coleslaw, Normal	▬	▬	▬																						

BOOTS

Coleslaw	▬	▬	▬																						
Apple, Peach & Nut Salad	▬	▬	▬	▬	▬																				
Chicken, Mushroom & Asparagus Salad	▬	▬	▬	▬																					
Tuna & Pasta Salad	▬	▬	▬	▬	▬																				

MARKS & SPENCER

Courgette, Pasta & Prawn Salad	▬	▬																							
Mexican Style Bean Salad	▬	▬																							
Carrot & Nut Salad	▬	▬	▬	▬																					

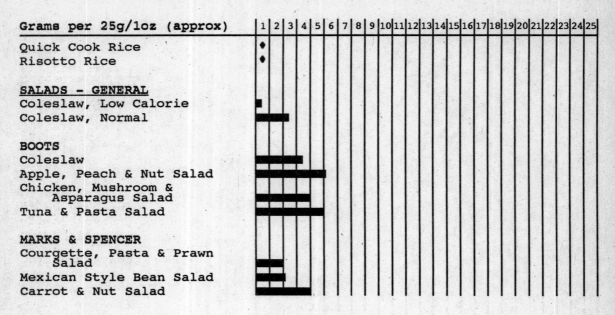

Cauliflower & Apple Salad
Cheese Coleslaw
Coleslaw
Florida Salad
Three Bean Salad

SAINSBURYS
Apple, Peach & Nut
Brown Rice Salad
Cheese Celery & Pineapple
    Salad
Crisp Vegetable Salad
Coleslaw
Coleslaw with Prawns
Coleslaw in Low Calorie
    Dressing
Celery, Apple & Mandarin
    Salad
Coleslaw in Mild Curried
    Dressing
Mild Curry Rice

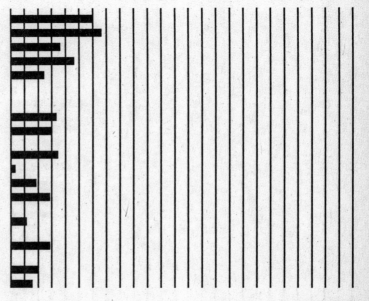

♦ = negligible

Grams per 25g/1oz (approx)	1	2	3	4	5	6	7	8	9	10	11	12	13	14	15	16	17	18	19	20	21	22	23	24	25

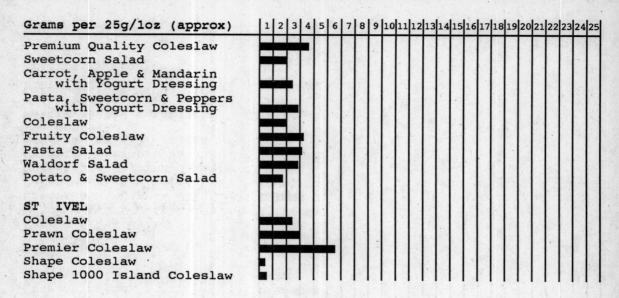

Premium Quality Coleslaw																									
Sweetcorn Salad																									
Carrot, Apple & Mandarin with Yogurt Dressing																									
Pasta, Sweetcorn & Peppers with Yogurt Dressing																									
Coleslaw																									
Fruity Coleslaw																									
Pasta Salad																									
Waldorf Salad																									
Potato & Sweetcorn Salad																									

ST IVEL

Coleslaw																									
Prawn Coleslaw																									
Premier Coleslaw																									
Shape Coleslaw																									
Shape 1000 Island Coleslaw																									

Shape Garlic and Herb
    Coleslaw
Shape Potato Salad
Shape Curried Potato Salad
Shape Chilli Potato Salad

TESCO
Broccoli Salad
Carrot & Nut Salad
Celery, Nut & Sultana Salad
Cheese & Pineapple Coleslaw
Coleslaw
Coronation Chicken Salad
Country Vegetable Salad
Fruit Coleslaw
Ham Coleslaw
Mediterranean Salad
Oriental Salad
Pasta & Tuna Salad
Pasta, Courgette & Prawn
    Salad

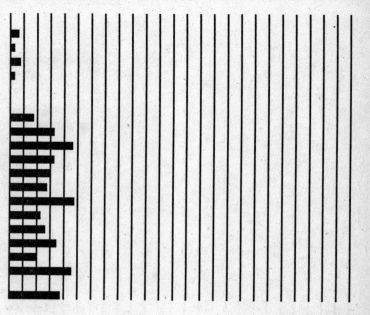

354

♦ = negligible

Grams per 25g/1oz (approx)

Food	Grams per 25g/1oz (approx)
Potato Salad	~6.5
Prawn Coleslaw	~2.5
Reduced Calorie Coleslaw	~1
Reduced Calorie Potato Salad	~1
Rice & Vegetable Salad	~1.5
Three Bean Salad	~2
WAITROSE	
American Pasta Salad	~1
Brown Rice Salad	~3.5
Cabbage & Walnut Salad	~2
Californian Salad	~3
Carnival Salad	~1.5
Carrot & Nut Salad	~6.5
Cauliflower & Broccoli Salad	~4
Chinese Leaf & Sweetcorn Salad	~1
Coleslaw	~3
Cottage Coleslaw	~7

Florida Salad
Harvest Salad with Orange
    Dressing
Leek & Bean Salad
Low Calorie Coleslaw
Mexican Bean Salad
Muesli Coleslaw
New Potato Salad
Pasta & Kababos Salad
Potato & Onion Salad
Potato & Chive Salad
Potato Salad with Mayonnaise
Potato & Frankfurter Salad
Prawn Salad
Sunrise Salad
Tabouleh Salad
Waldorf Salad
Wild Rice salad
Winter Salad

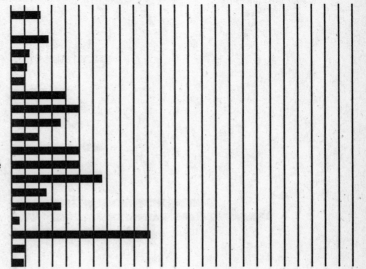

♦ = negligible

356

Grams per 25g/1oz (approx)	1	2	3	4	5	6	7	8	9	10	11	12	13	14	15	16	17	18	19	20	21	22	23	24	25

SAVOURY SAUCES, DRESSINGS & PACKET MIXES - GENERAL

Item	Grams per 25g/1oz (approx)
1000 Island Dressing	9
Bread Sauce	2
Brown Sauce	1
Cheese Sauce	4
French Dressing	20
Mayonnaise	15
Onion Sauce	—
Salad Cream	7
Waistline	4
Seafood Dressing - non diet	7
Tomato Ketchup	1
Tomato Purée	1
Tomato Sauce	2
White Sauce - Savoury	3

357

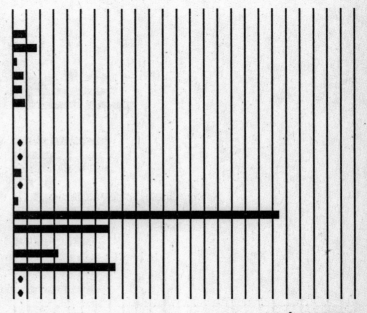

CAMPBELLS
Pizza Topping Sauce
Bolognese
Sauce for Bolognese
Tomato & Mushroom Sauce
Siciliana Sauce
Bolognese Sauce

CO-OP
Brown Sauce
Fruity Sauce
Horseradish Sauce
Mint Sauce
Piccalilli Sauce
Mayonnaise
Reduced Calorie Mayonnaise
Reduced Calorie Vinegar &
    Oil Dressing
Salad Cream
Tomato Ketchup
Tomato Puree - Can/Tube/Jar

♦ = negligible

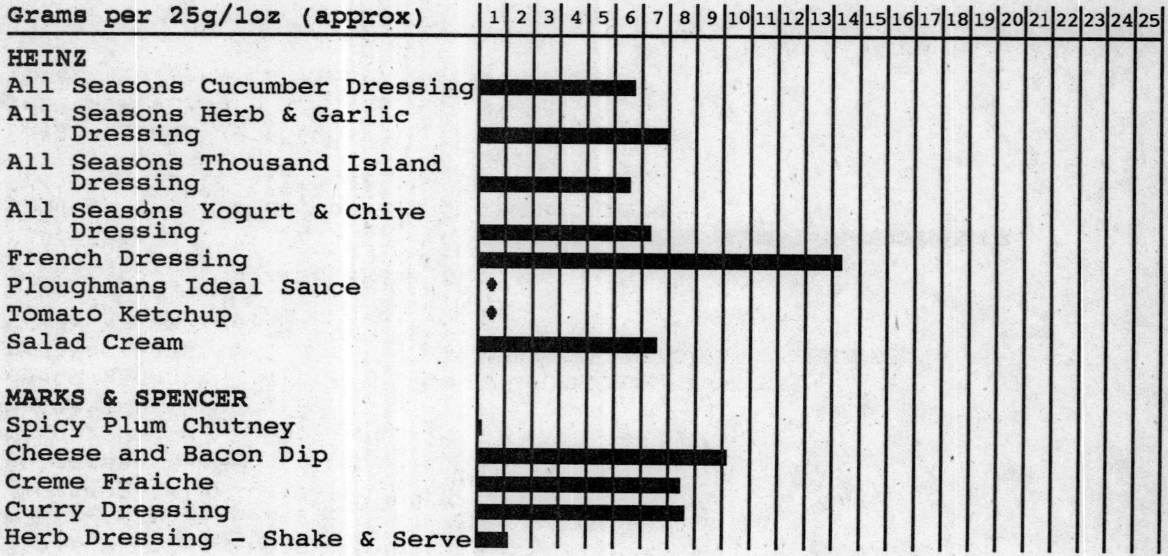

Grams per 25g/1oz (approx)	1	2	3	4	5	6	7	8	9	10	11	12	13	14	15	16	17	18	19	20	21	22	23	24	25

HEINZ

All Seasons Cucumber Dressing	6
All Seasons Herb & Garlic Dressing	7
All Seasons Thousand Island Dressing	6
All Seasons Yogurt & Chive Dressing	7
French Dressing	13.5
Ploughmans Ideal Sauce	•
Tomato Ketchup	•
Salad Cream	7

MARKS & SPENCER

Spicy Plum Chutney	
Cheese and Bacon Dip	9.5
Creme Fraiche	7.5
Curry Dressing	7.5
Herb Dressing – Shake & Serve	0.5

359

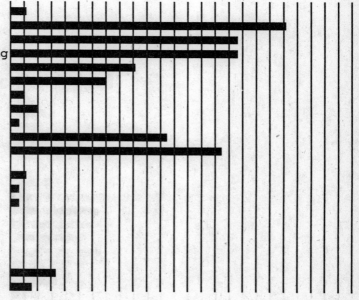

Herb Salad Dressing
Marie Rose Dressing
Mayonnaise – Fresh
Shake & Serve French Dressing
Sour Cream Dressing – Onion
Thousand Island Dressing
Bolognese Sauce
Mornay Sauce
Napoletana Sauce
Pesto Sauce
Tartare Sauce
Cream & Mushroom Cooking
    Sauce
Sweet & Sour Cooking Sauce
Red Wine Cooking Sauce

NESTLE (Crosse & Blackwell)

Dish of the Day (Sachets)
Barbecue Style
Barbecue Glaze

♦ = negligible

360

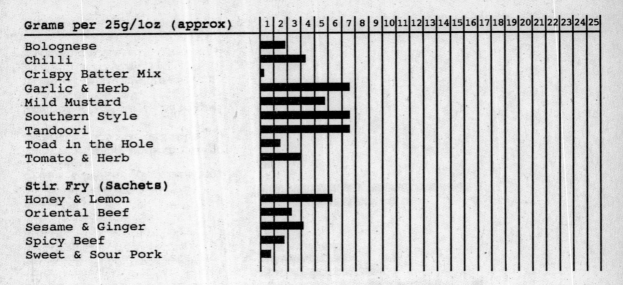

Grams per 25g/1oz (approx)	1	2	3	4	5	6	7	8	9	10	11	12	13	14	15	16	17	18	19	20	21	22	23	24	25
Bolognese		▮																							
Chilli			▮																						
Crispy Batter Mix	▮																								
Garlic & Herb							▮																		
Mild Mustard					▮																				
Southern Style							▮																		
Tandoori							▮																		
Toad in the Hole	▮																								
Tomato & Herb			▮																						
Stir Fry (Sachets)																									
Honey & Lemon						▮																			
Oriental Beef		▮																							
Sesame & Ginger			▮																						
Spicy Beef		▮																							
Sweet & Sour Pork	▮																								

361

Bonne Cuisine Sauces
(Sachets)
Au Poivre
Bolognese
Hollandaise Sauce
Madeira Wine Gravy
Mature Cheddar Sauce
Onion with White Wine Sauce
White Wine Sauce

Cook in Pot - Canned
Hong Kong
Shanghai
Spare Rib
Sweet & Sour

Sauces
Branston Fruity
Branston Spicy
Tomato Ketchup
Healthy Balance Ketchup

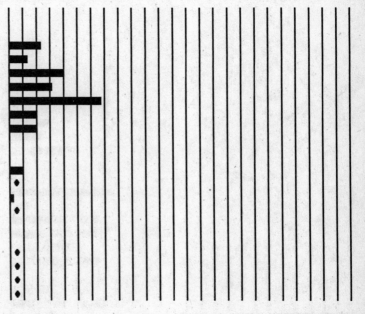

◆ = negligible

362

Grams per 25g/1oz (approx)	Value
Salad Cream (Sunflower Oil)	9
Waistline Range of Dressings	
Oil Free French Dressing	◆
Oil Free Vinaigrette	◆
Vinegar & Oil Dressing	3
Tomato Dressing	2½
Tomato Ketchup	◆
Reduced Oil Mayonnaise	8
Cook in the Pot - Dry Mixes	
Barbecue Chicken	2½
Beef Goulash	3
Beef Stroganoff	3½
Chicken Chasseur	3
Chicken Provencale	3
Chilli Con Carne	3½
Fish Bonne Femme	2
Lamb Ragout	2½

Madras Curry
Moussaka
Sausage & Tomato Casserole
Shepherds Pie
Steak & Kidney

SAINSBURYS
Bolognese Sauce
Brown Sauce
Carbonara Sauce
Chilli Sauce – Canned
Classic Italian Sauce
Cranberry Sauce
Creamed Horseradish Sauce
Fresh Garden Mint
Fruit Sauce
Horseradish Sauce
Italian Tomato Ketchup
Mint Jelly
Napoletana Sauce
Provencale Sauce – Canned

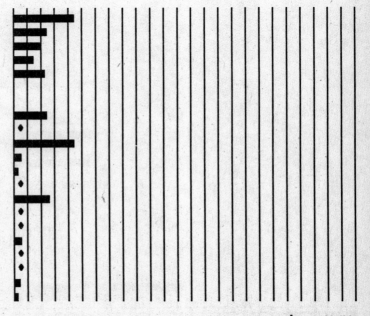

◆ = negligible

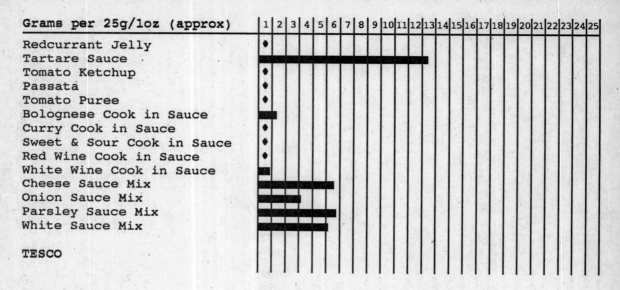

Grams per 25g/1oz (approx)	1	2	3	4	5	6	7	8	9	10	11	12	13	14	15	16	17	18	19	20	21	22	23	24	25
Redcurrant Jelly																									
Tartare Sauce																									
Tomato Ketchup																									
Passata																									
Tomato Puree																									
Bolognese Cook in Sauce																									
Curry Cook in Sauce																									
Sweet & Sour Cook in Sauce																									
Red Wine Cook in Sauce																									
White Wine Cook in Sauce																									
Cheese Sauce Mix																									
Onion Sauce Mix																									
Parsley Sauce Mix																									
White Sauce Mix																									

TESCO

365

Dry
Bread Sauce
Beef Stroganoff
Cheese Sauce
Chicken Chasseur
Chilli Con Carne
Curry Sauce
Goulash
Madras Curry
Onion Sauce
Parsley Sauce
Savoury White Sauce

Bottled
Brown Sauce
Economy Brown Sauce
Economy Tomato Ketchup
Fruit Sauce
Spicy Brown Sauce
Tomato Ketchup
Traditional Brown Sauce

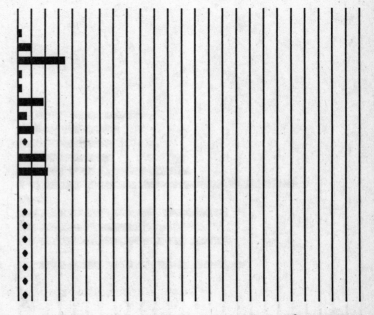

♦ = negligible

366

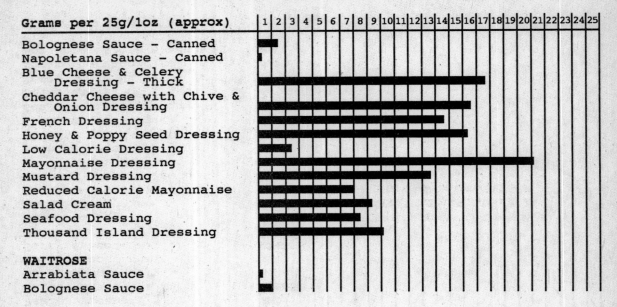

Grams per 25g/1oz (approx)	1	2	3	4	5	6	7	8	9	10	11	12	13	14	15	16	17	18	19	20	21	22	23	24	25
Bolognese Sauce – Canned																									
Napoletana Sauce – Canned																									
Blue Cheese & Celery Dressing – Thick																									
Cheddar Cheese with Chive & Onion Dressing																									
French Dressing																									
Honey & Poppy Seed Dressing																									
Low Calorie Dressing																									
Mayonnaise Dressing																									
Mustard Dressing																									
Reduced Calorie Mayonnaise																									
Salad Cream																									
Seafood Dressing																									
Thousand Island Dressing																									
WAITROSE																									
Arrabiata Sauce																									
Bolognese Sauce																									

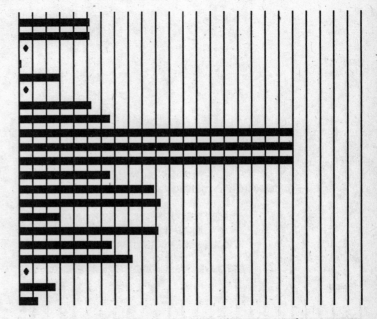

Carbonara Sauce
Cheese Sauce
Fruit Sauce
Napoletana Sauce
Sate Sauce
Spicy Sauce
Tartare Sauce
Salad Cream
Mayonnaise
Lemon Mayonnaise
Garlic Mayonnaise
Reduced Calorie Mayonnaise
Blue Cheese Dressing
French Dressing
Low/Cal Vin & Oil Dressing
Italian Dressing
Seafood Dressing
Thousand Island Dressing
Tomato Ketchup
Creamed Horseradish
Hot Horseradish Sauce

♦ = negligible

368

Grams per 25g/1oz (approx)	1	2	3	4	5	6	7	8	9	10	11	12	13	14	15	16	17	18	19	20	21	22	23	24	25
Horseradish Relish	■																								

SLIMMERS PRODUCTS

BOOTS

	1	2	3	4	5	6	7	8	9	10	11	12	13	14	15	16	17	18	19	20	21	22	23	24	25
Chicken Noodle Snack Soup	♦																								
Low Calorie Mayonnaise	██████████																								
Low Calorie Sweet Pickle	♦																								
Mushroom Snack Soup	■																								
New Beef Oriental Ready Meal	■																								
New Chicken Curry Ready Meal	■																								
New Chicken Supreme Ready Meal	■																								
Sharp Low Calorie Lemon Juice	♦																								
Tropical Fruit Low Calorie Drink	♦																								
New Paprika Beef Casserole	■																								
Tuna & Pasta Bake Ready Meal	■																								

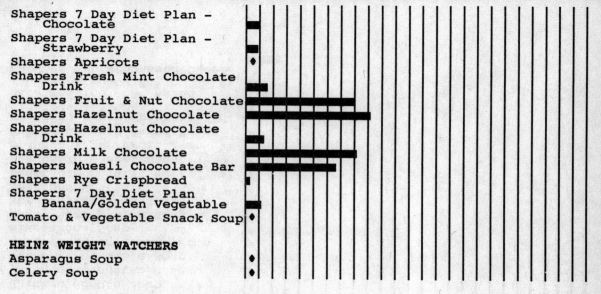

Shapers 7 Day Diet Plan – Chocolate

Shapers 7 Day Diet Plan – Strawberry

Shapers Apricots

Shapers Fresh Mint Chocolate Drink

Shapers Fruit & Nut Chocolate

Shapers Hazelnut Chocolate

Shapers Hazelnut Chocolate Drink

Shapers Milk Chocolate

Shapers Muesli Chocolate Bar

Shapers Rye Crispbread

Shapers 7 Day Diet Plan Banana/Golden Vegetable

Tomato & Vegetable Snack Soup

HEINZ WEIGHT WATCHERS
Asparagus Soup
Celery Soup

370

♦ = negligible

Grams per 25g/1oz (approx)

	1	2	3	4	5	6	7	8	9	10	11	12	13	14	15	16	17	18	19	20	21	22	23	24	25
Chicken Soup	♦																								
Chicken Noodle Soup	♦																								
Chicken & Vegetable Soup	♦																								
Country Vegetable Soup	♦																								
Mediterranean Tomato Soup	♦																								
Minestrone Soup	♦																								
Spicy Beef & Rice Soup	♦																								
Spring Vegetable Soup	♦																								
Tomato Soup	♦																								
Vegetable Soup	♦																								
Vegetable & Beef Soup	♦																								
Reduced Sugar Fruit Jams	♦																								
No Added Sugar Baked Beans	♦																								
No Added Sugar Spaghetti in Tomato Sauce	♦																								
Rice Pudding – No Added Sugar – Low Fat	▮																								
Reduced Fat Processed Cheese Slices	███																								

Reduced Fat Hard Cheese
Reduced Calorie Dressing
Reduced Calorie Mayonnaise
Sliced White Bread
Sliced Brown Bread
White Bread Rolls
Brown Bread Rolls
Danish White Loaf
Danish Brown Loaf
Reduced Calorie Ice Cream
Reduced Calorie Neapolitan
    Ice Cream

Menu Plus Range
Beef Oriental with Special
    Egg Rice
Chicken in Chinese Sauce
    with Rice
Chicken in Supreme Sauce
    with Vegetables

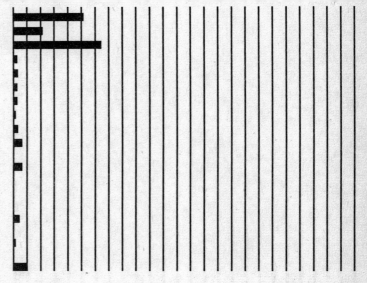

♦ = negligible

Grams per 25g/1oz (approx)	1	2	3	4	5	6	7	8	9	10	11	12	13	14	15	16	17	18	19	20	21	22	23	24	25
Prawn Provencale with Piquant Rice																									
Salmon Mornay with Broccoli																									
Vegetable Plus Range																									
Vegetable Au Gratin																									
Vegetable Curry																									
Vegetable Lasagne																									
Vegetable Moussaka																									
Pasta Plus Range																									
Beef Lasagne																									
Chicken & Ham Cacciatore																									
Pasta Shells with Vegetables & Prawns																									
Spaghetti Bolognese																									

373

SOUPS - GENERAL
Bone & Vegetable Broth
Chicken Cream of:
Ready to Serve
Condensed
Condensed, as served
Chicken Noodle
Lentil
Minestrone
Mushroom, Cream of
Oxtail
Tomato, Cream of:
Ready to Serve
Condensed
Condensed, as served
Vegetable

BATCHELORS

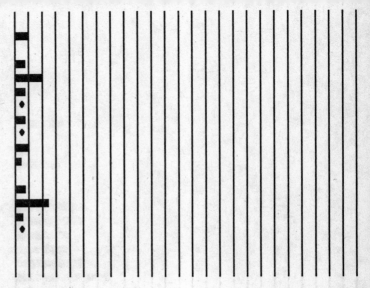

= negligible

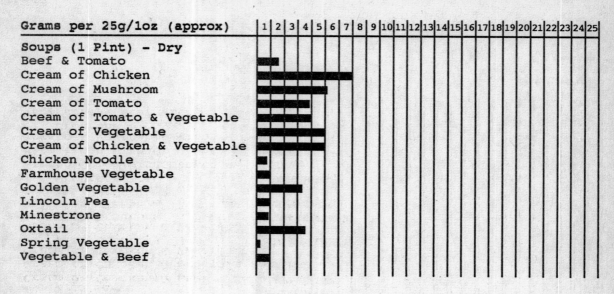

Grams per 25g/1oz (approx)	1	2	3	4	5	6	7	8	9	10	11	12	13	14	15	16	17	18	19	20	21	22	23	24	25

Soups (1 Pint) - Dry

Beef & Tomato
Cream of Chicken
Cream of Mushroom
Cream of Tomato
Cream of Tomato & Vegetable
Cream of Vegetable
Cream of Chicken & Vegetable
Chicken Noodle
Farmhouse Vegetable
Golden Vegetable
Lincoln Pea
Minestrone
Oxtail
Spring Vegetable
Vegetable & Beef

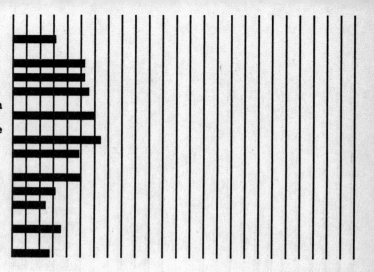

No Simmer Soups
Beef & Tomato with Croutons
Cream of Asparagus with Croutons
Cream of Chicken & Leek
Cream of Chicken & Mushroom
Cream of Chicken & Sweetcorn with Croutons
Cream of Chicken & Vegetable with Croutons
Cream of Mushroom
Cream of Vegetable with Croutons
French Onion with Croutons
Minestrone with Croutons
Tomato & Vegetable with Croutons
Vegetable & Beef with Croutons

◆ = negligible

376

Grams per 25g/1oz (approx)	1	2	3	4	5	6	7	8	9	10	11	12	13	14	15	16	17	18	19	20	21	22	23	24	25
Slim-A-Soup																									
Beef & Tomato	◆																								
Beef & Vegetable	▮																								
Chicken & Vegetable	◆																								
Chicken & Sweetcorn	▮																								
Chicken	◆																								
Chicken & Leek	◆																								
Chicken Noodle	◆																								
Clear Chicken with Crouton	▮																								
Clear Beef with Croutons	▮																								
Golden Vegetable	◆																								
Minestrone	◆																								
Tomato & Vegetable	▮																								
Vegetable & Beef	◆																								

CAMPBELLS

377

Gourmet Soups Condensed
Chicken & Sweetcorn
Crab Bisque
Cream of Asparagus
Cream of Broccoli
Cream of Smoked Salmon
French Onion
Goulash

Condensed Soups
Beef Broth
Chicken Noodle
Chicken Rice
Consomme
Cream of Celery
Cream of Chicken
Cream of Mushroom
Cream of Potato & Leek
Cream of Tomato
Golden Vegetable
Irish Broth

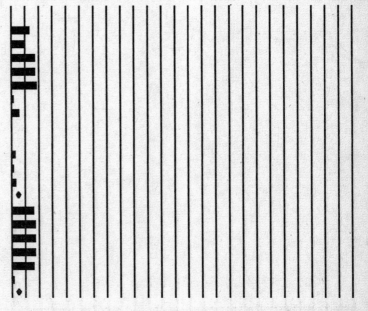

♦ = negligible

Grams per 25g/1oz (approx)	1	2	3	4	5	6	7	8	9	10	11	12	13	14	15	16	17	18	19	20	21	22	23	24	25
Lentil																									
Minestrone																									
Mulligatawny																									
Ox Tail																									
Oxtail & Vegetable																									
Pea & Ham																									
Scotch Broth																									
Tomato																									
Tomato Rice																									
Turkey & Vegetable Broth																									
Vegetable																									
Main Course Soups – Ready to Serve																									
Beef & Vegetable																									
Chicken & Vegetable																									
Chilli Con Carne																									
Steak, Kidney & Vegetable																									
Steak & Potato																									

Grannys Soups
Chicken & Vegetable Broth
    with Rice
Cream of Chicken
Cream of Potato
Cream of Tomato
Lentil
Mushroom
Potato & Leek
Scotch Broth
Tomato
Vegetable
Winter Vegetable

Bumper Harvest Soups
Cream of Chicken
Cream of Mushroom
Cream of Tomato
Lentil
Minestrone
Ox Tail

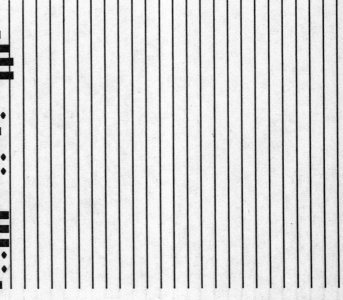

♦ = negligible

380

Grams per 25g/1oz (approx)	1	2	3	4	5	6	7	8	9	10	11	12	13	14	15	16	17	18	19	20	21	22	23	24	25
Scotch Broth																									
Vegetable																									
Soup In Glass																									
Beef with Waterchestnut																									
Chicken Tarragon																									
Chicken Tikka																									
Prawn Bisque																									
Tomato Italienne																									
CO-OP																									
Celery - Creamed																									
Chicken - Creamed																									
Chicken & Mushroom - Creamed																									
French Onion																									
Golden Vegetable																									
Lentil																									
Minestrone																									
Mushroom - Creamed																									

381

Oxtail
Pea & Ham
Potato & Leek
Scotch Broth
Thick Vegetable
Tomato – Creamed
Vegetable
Vegetable & Beef

HEINZ

Ready to Serve Soups
Beef Soup
Cream of Celery
Cream of Chicken
Golden Chicken & Mushroom
Golden Vegetable
Homestyle Country Vegetable
Invaders – Cream of Tomato
    with Pasta Shapes
Minestrone

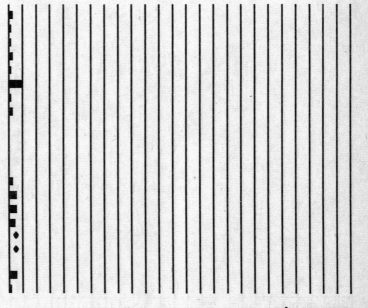

♦ = negligible

Grams per 25g/1oz (approx)	1	2	3	4	5	6	7	8	9	10	11	12	13	14	15	16	17	18	19	20	21	22	23	24	25
Big Soups																									
Beef & Vegetable	♦																								
Beef Broth	♦																								
Chicken & Vegetable	▌																								
Golden Vegetable	♦																								
Vegetable	♦																								
Special Recipe Soups																									
Cream of Asparagus	■																								
Cream of Chicken with White Wine	■																								
Cock-a-Leekie	♦																								
Game	♦																								
Farmhouse Soups																									
Beef & Vegetable	♦																								
Beef Broth	♦																								
Chicken & Vegetable	♦																								
Cream of Tomato	■																								

383

Cream of Mushroom
Oxtail
Potato & Leek
Scotch Broth
Scottish Vegetable with
    Lentils
Spring Vegetable
Vegetable

Whole Soups
Farmhouse Vegetable
Lentil
Pea & Ham
Tomato & Lentil
Winter Vegetable

Spicy Soups
Curried Chicken with Rice
Chilli Bean & Beef
Mulligatawny
Tomato & Green Pepper

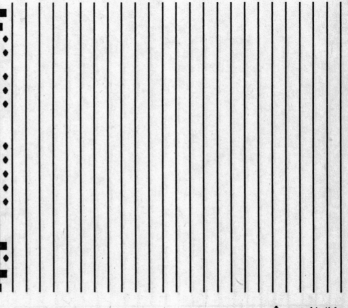

♦ = negligible

Grams per 25g/1oz (approx)	1	2	3	4	5	6	7	8	9	10	11	12	13	14	15	16	17	18	19	20	21	22	23	24	25

MARKS & SPENCER

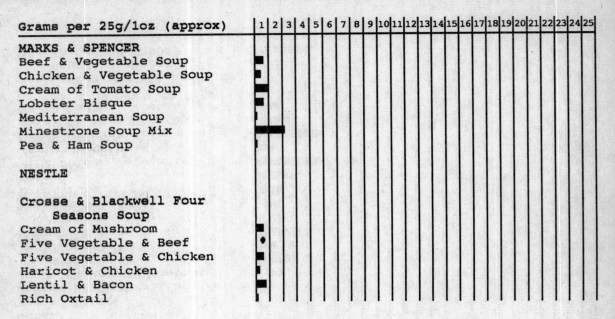

Beef & Vegetable Soup
Chicken & Vegetable Soup
Cream of Tomato Soup
Lobster Bisque
Mediterranean Soup
Minestrone Soup Mix
Pea & Ham Soup

NESTLE

Crosse & Blackwell Four Seasons Soup
Cream of Mushroom
Five Vegetable & Beef
Five Vegetable & Chicken
Haricot & Chicken
Lentil & Bacon
Rich Oxtail

Rich Tomato
Spicy Beef & Tomato

Crosse & Blackwell Box Soups
Beef Flavour & Vegetable
Chicken & Leek
Chicken Noodle
Country Mushroom
Country Tomato
Farmers Thick Onion
Minestrone
Oxtail
Rick Golden Vegetable
Spring Vegetable
Thick Chicken
Thick Country Vegetable
Thick Garden Vegetable

**Crosse & Blackwell No Simmer
    Soups (Sachets)**
Asparagus & Mushroom

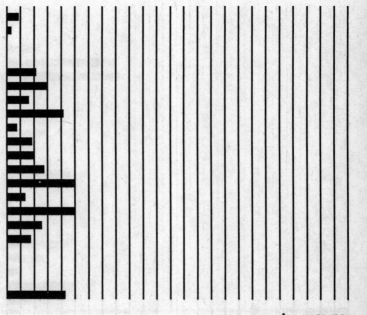

♦ = negligible

386

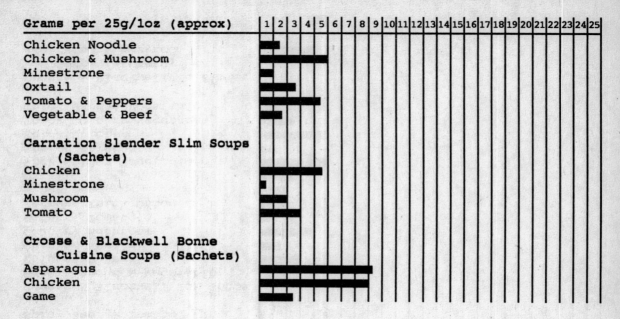

Grams per 25g/1oz (approx)	1	2	3	4	5	6	7	8	9	10	11	12	13	14	15	16	17	18	19	20	21	22	23	24	25
Chicken Noodle																									
Chicken & Mushroom																									
Minestrone																									
Oxtail																									
Tomato & Peppers																									
Vegetable & Beef																									
Carnation Slender Slim Soups (Sachets)																									
Chicken																									
Minestrone																									
Mushroom																									
Tomato																									
Crosse & Blackwell Bonne Cuisine Soups (Sachets)																									
Asparagus																									
Chicken																									
Game																									

387

Lobster Bisque
Mushroom
Vegetable

**Crosse & Blackwell Canned
    Soup**
Cream of Chicken
Cream of Mushroom
Cream of Tomato
Consomme
Garden Vegetable
Harvest Thick Vegetable
Oxtail
Scotch Broth
Scottish Lentil
Vichyssoise

Chunky Soups
Beef & Vegetable
Chicken & Vegetable
Tomato & Vegetable

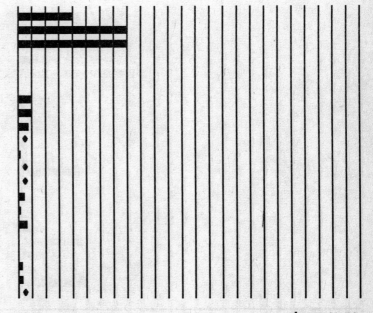

♦ = negligible

Grams per 25g/1oz (approx)	1	2	3	4	5	6	7	8	9	10	11	12	13	14	15	16	17	18	19	20	21	22	23	24	25
Vegetable	♦																								
TESCO																									
Canned																									
Cream of Celery																									
Cream of Chicken																									
Cream of Mushroom																									
Cream of Tomato																									
Lentil																									
Minestrone																									
Oxtail																									
Scotch Broth																									
Thick Vegetable																									
Vegetable																									
Dry Mix																									
Chicken Noodle																									
Cream of Asparagus																									

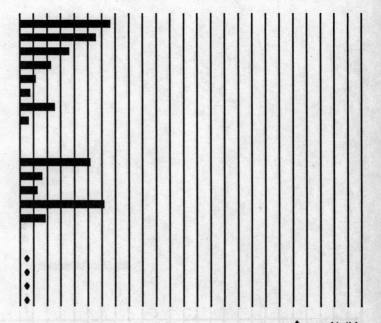

Cream of Chicken
Cream of Mushroom
Cream of Tomato
French Onion
Minestrone
Oxtail
Spring Vegetable
Vegetable & Beef

Instant (Dry Mix)
Chicken & Vegetable
French Onion
Minestrone
Thick Mushroom
Tomato and Vegetable

WAITROSE
Low/Cal Asparagus
Low/Cal Celery
Low/Cal Chicken/Vegetable
Low/Cal Mushroom

♦ = negligible

Grams per 25g/1oz (approx)

Soup	Grams per 25g/1oz (approx)
Low/Cal Tomato	1
Low/Cal Tomato/Beef	1
Low/Cal Vegetable	1
Asparagus Quick Soup	8
Beef Broth	1
Beef Consomme	1
Chicken & Sweetcorn	1
Chicken	
Chicken & Leek	2
Chicken & Mushroom Quick	3
Chicken & Veg Quick Soup	4
Chicken Noodle	1
Clam Chowder	1
Cock-a-Leekie	1
Crab Bisque	1
Cream of Celery	1
Cream of Asparagus	1
Cream of Veg Quick Soup	4
Cream of Tomato	1

French Onion
Goulash
Lentil & Bacon
Lobster Bisque
Minestrone
Minestrone Quick Soup
Mushroom
Oxtail
Pea & Ham
Scotch Broth
Spring Vegetable
Tomato & Veg Quick Soup
Vegetable
Vichyssoise

SPREADS, PATES & PASTES

CO-OP
Beef & Ham Paste
Chicken & Ham Paste
Salmon & Shrimp Paste

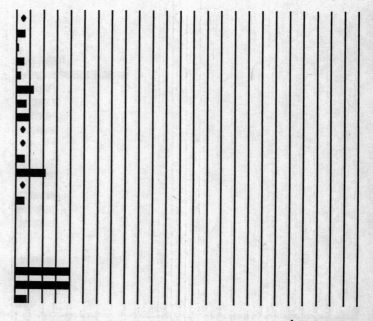

♦ = negligible

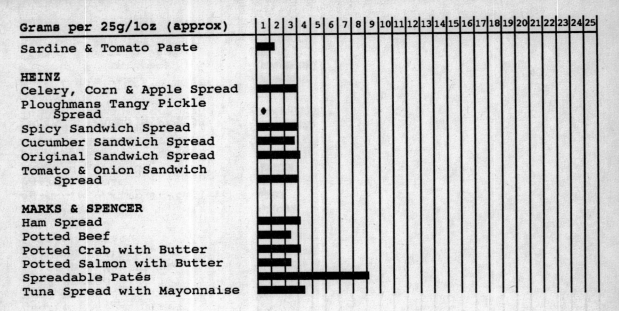

Grams per 25g/1oz (approx)	1	2	3	4	5	6	7	8	9	10	11	12	13	14	15	16	17	18	19	20	21	22	23	24	25

Sardine & Tomato Paste

HEINZ
Celery, Corn & Apple Spread
Ploughmans Tangy Pickle
    Spread
Spicy Sandwich Spread
Cucumber Sandwich Spread
Original Sandwich Spread
Tomato & Onion Sandwich
    Spread

MARKS & SPENCER
Ham Spread
Potted Beef
Potted Crab with Butter
Potted Salmon with Butter
Spreadable Patés
Tuna Spread with Mayonnaise

393

SAINSBURYS

Pastes & Spreads
Beef & Onion Spread
Beef Paste
Beef Spread
Chicken & Ham Paste
Chicken Paste
Chicken Spread
Crab Spread
Crab Paste
Salmon & Shrimp Paste
Salmon Spread
Sandwich Spread
Sardine & Tomato Spread
Sardine & Tomato Paste
Tuna & Mayonnaise Paste
Tuna & Mayonnaise Spread

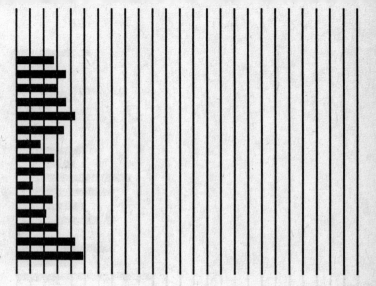

394

◆ = negligible

Grams per 25g/1oz (approx)	1	2	3	4	5	6	7	8	9	10	11	12	13	14	15	16	17	18	19	20	21	22	23	24	25

Paté

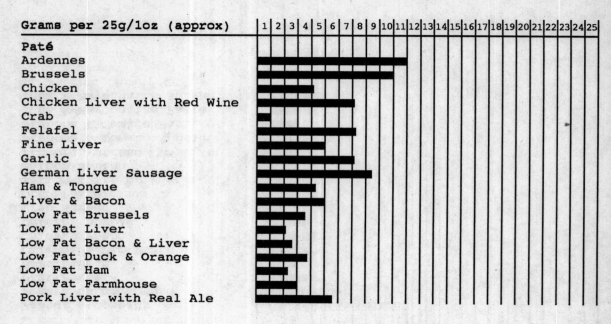

Paté	Grams
Ardennes	11
Brussels	10
Chicken	4.5
Chicken Liver with Red Wine	7
Crab	1
Felafel	7.5
Fine Liver	5
Garlic	7
German Liver Sausage	9.5
Ham & Tongue	4.5
Liver & Bacon	5
Low Fat Brussels	4
Low Fat Liver	3
Low Fat Bacon & Liver	2.5
Low Fat Duck & Orange	3.5
Low Fat Ham	2.5
Low Fat Farmhouse	2.5
Pork Liver with Real Ale	5.5

Provencale
Sliced German Liver Sausage
Smoked Mackerel
Smoked Salmon
Turkey & Ham
Vegetable
Vegetable Terrine

TESCO

Pastes & Spreads
Beef Paste
Beef Spread
Chicken and Ham Spread
Chicken Paste
Chicken Spread
Crab Paste
Crab Spread
Salmon and Shrimp Paste
Salmon Spread
Sandwich Spread

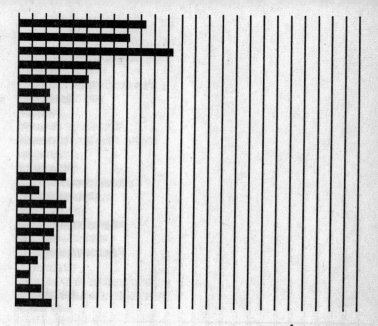

◆ = negligible

Grams per 25g/1oz (approx)	1	2	3	4	5	6	7	8	9	10	11	12	13	14	15	16	17	18	19	20	21	22	23	24	25

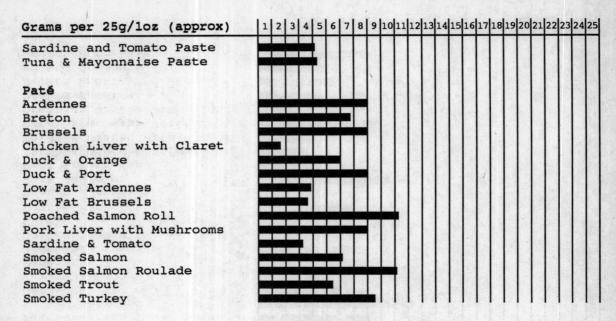

	Grams per 25g/1oz (approx)
Sardine and Tomato Paste	4½
Tuna & Mayonnaise Paste	4½
Paté	
Ardennes	8½
Breton	7
Brussels	8
Chicken Liver with Claret	6½
Duck & Orange	6½
Duck & Port	7½
Low Fat Ardennes	4½
Low Fat Brussels	4½
Poached Salmon Roll	11
Pork Liver with Mushrooms	8
Sardine & Tomato	3½
Smoked Salmon	6½
Smoked Salmon Roulade	11
Smoked Trout	5½
Smoked Turkey	9½

Tuna
Vegetable

WAITROSE

Paté
Ardennes
Chicken Red Wine
Chicken
Coarse Pork Liver
Crab
Duck Supreme
Duck & Port Wine
Farmhouse Low Fat
Norfolk Coarse with Ale
Pork Liver with Veal
Scottish Garlic with Brandy
Smoked Mackerel
Smoked Trout
Smoked Salmon
Smooth Pork Liver

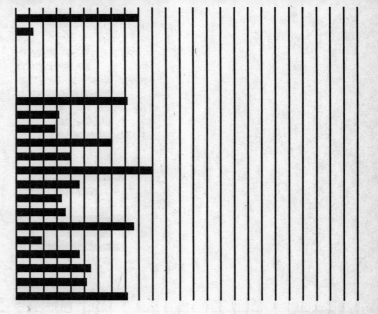

♦ = negligible

Grams per 25g/1oz (approx)	1	2	3	4	5	6	7	8	9	10	11	12	13	14	15	16	17	18	19	20	21	22	23	24	25
Tuna																									
Venison with Burgundy Wine																									

SOYA – GENERAL

| Soya, full fat | | | | | | | | | | | | | | | | | | | | | | | | | |
| Soya, low fat | | | | | | | | | | | | | | | | | | | | | | | | | |

DIETBURGER COMPANY LIMITED

| Dietburger | | | | | | | | | | | | | | | | | | | | | | | | | |

SUGARS – GENERAL

Glucose Liquid																									
Sugar																									
Syrup																									
Treacle																									

BOOTS

| Saccharin Tablets | | | | | | | | | | | | | | | | | | | | | | | | | |
| Sugar Lite | | | | | | | | | | | | | | | | | | | | | | | | | |

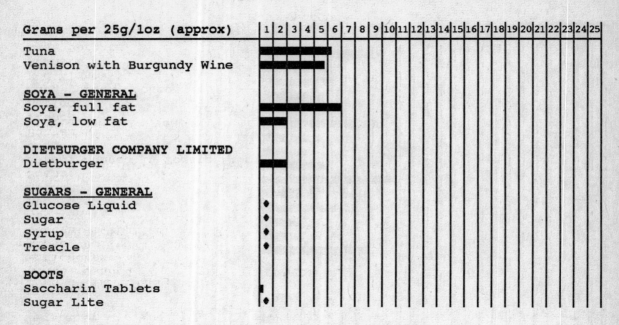

399

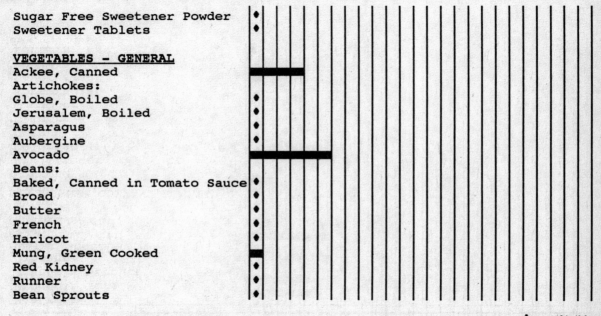

Sugar Free Sweetener Powder	♦	
Sweetener Tablets	♦	
VEGETABLES – GENERAL		
Ackee, Canned	▬▬▬▬	
Artichokes:		
Globe, Boiled	♦	
Jerusalem, Boiled	♦	
Asparagus	♦	
Aubergine	♦	
Avocado	▬▬▬▬▬▬	
Beans:		
Baked, Canned in Tomato Sauce	♦	
Broad	♦	
Butter	♦	
French	♦	
Haricot	♦	
Mung, Green Cooked	▬	
Red Kidney	♦	
Runner	♦	
Bean Sprouts	♦	

400

♦ = negligible

Grams per 25g/1oz (approx)	1	2	3	4	5	6	7	8	9	10	11	12	13	14	15	16	17	18	19	20	21	22	23	24	25
Beetroot	◆																								
Broccoli Tops	◆																								
Brussels Sprouts	◆																								
Cabbage:																									
Red	◆																								
Savoy	◆																								
Spring	◆																								
White	◆																								
Winter	◆																								
Carrots	◆																								
Cauliflower	◆																								
Celeriac	◆																								
Celery	◆																								
Chicory	◆																								
Cucumber	◆																								
Horseradish	◆																								
Laverbread	■																								
Leeks	◆																								
Lentils, Raw	■																								

Masar Dhal, Cooked	
Lettuce	♦
Marrow	♦
Mushrooms, Raw	♦
Mushrooms, Fried	
Mustard & Cress	♦
Okra	♦
Onions, all except Fried	♦
Onions, Fried	
Parsley	♦
Parsnips	♦
Peas, all kinds	♦
Chick Peas:	
Bengal, Cooked Dhal	
Channa, Dhal	
Peppers, Green	♦
Plantain:	
Green, Boiled	♦
Ripe, Fried	

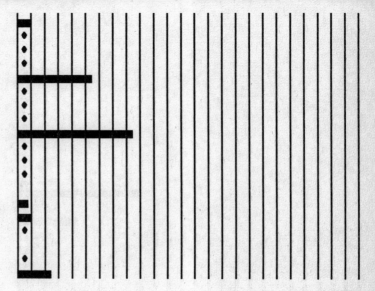

402

♦ = negligible

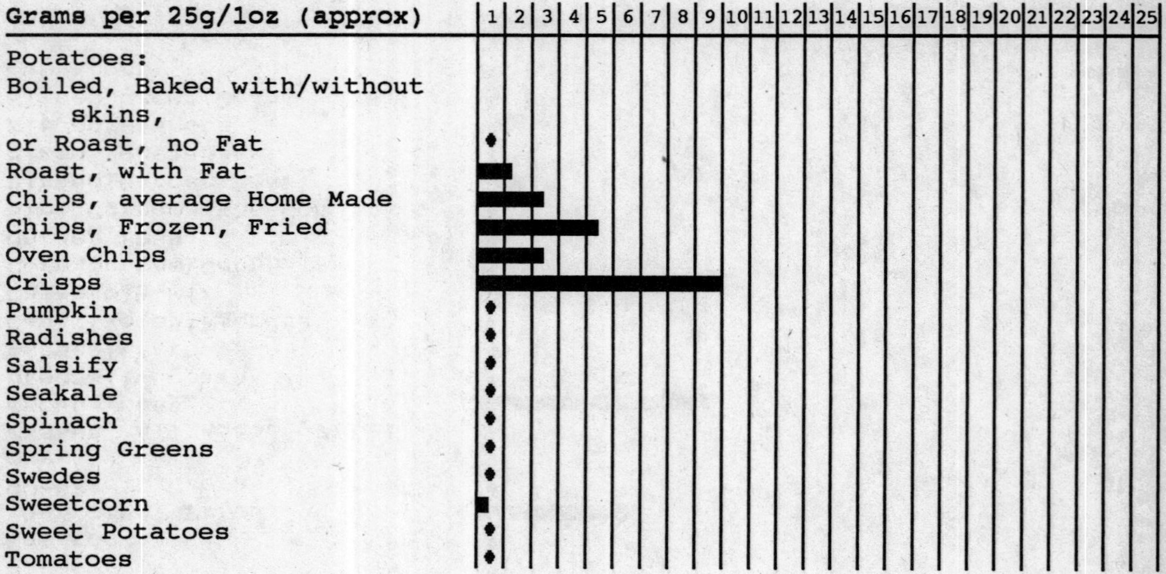

Grams per 25g/1oz (approx)	1	2	3	4	5	6	7	8	9	10	11	12	13	14	15	16	17	18	19	20	21	22	23	24	25

Potatoes:
Boiled, Baked with/without skins, or Roast, no Fat ▪

Roast, with Fat ▬

Chips, average Home Made ▬▬

Chips, Frozen, Fried ▬▬▬▬

Oven Chips ▬▬

Crisps ▬▬▬▬▬▬▬▬▬

Pumpkin ▪

Radishes ▪

Salsify ▪

Seakale ▪

Spinach ▪

Spring Greens ▪

Swedes ▪

Sweetcorn ▬

Sweet Potatoes ▪

Tomatoes ▪

403

Tomatoes, Fried
Turnips
Watercress
Yam

CO-OP

Frozen
Broad Beans
Broccoli Spears
Brussel Sprouts
Cauliflower Florets
Casserole Mix
Corn on the Cob
Garden Peas
Mini Corn on the Cob
Minted Garden Peas
Mixed Vegetables
Sliced Carrots
Sliced Green Beans
Sweetcorn

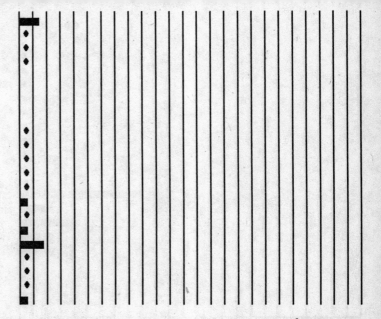

♦ = negligible

Grams per 25g/1oz (approx)	1	2	3	4	5	6	7	8	9	10	11	12	13	14	15	16	17	18	19	20	21	22	23	24	25
Whole Small Carrots	◆																								
Value Garden Peas	◆																								
Chunky Chips	■																								
Crinkle Cut Chips	■																								
Straight Cut Chips	■																								
Oven Chips	▬																								
Potato Croquettes	◆																								
Potato Waffles	▬▬																								
Canned																									
Broad Beans	◆																								
Butter Beans	◆																								
Cut Green Beans	◆																								
Garden Peas	◆																								
Italian Chopped Tomatoes	◆																								
Italian Peeled Tomatoes	◆																								
Jersey New Potatoes	◆																								
Marrowfat Processed Peas	◆																								
Mixed Vegetables	◆																								

Mushy Processed Peas ♦
New Potatoes ♦
Red Kidney Beans ♦
Sliced Carrots ♦
Sliced Green Beans ♦
Small Grilling Mushrooms ♦
Small Processed Peas ♦
Sweetcorn |
Sweetcorn with Peppers |
Whole Carrots ♦
Garden Peas – No Added Salt ♦
Sliced Carrots – No Added
     Salt ♦
Sliced Green Beans – No
     Added Salt ♦
Sweetcorn – No Added Salt |
Whole Carrots – No Added Salt ♦

ICELAND
Economy Peas ♦
Minted Peas ♦

♦ = negligible

Grams per 25g/1oz (approx)	1	2	3	4	5	6	7	8	9	10	11	12	13	14	15	16	17	18	19	20	21	22	23	24	25
Garden Peas	◆																								
Mushy Peas	◆																								
Petit Pois	◆																								
Mange Tout	◆																								
Sliced Green Beans	◆																								
Whole Green Beans	◆																								
Cut Green Beans	◆																								
Broad Beans	▮																								
Very Fine Whole Beans	◆																								
Baby Carrots	◆																								
Diced Carrots	◆																								
Sliced Carrots	◆																								
Julienne Carrots	◆																								
Baby Cobs of Corn	◆																								
Mini Cobs	▮																								
Crinkle Cut Oven Chips	███																								
Steak Cut Chips	███																								
Straight Cut Chips	███																								
Crinkle Cut Chips	███																								

407

Slim Fries
Potato Croquettes
Potato Nuggets
Jacket Wedges
Roast Potatoes
Brussels Sprouts
Button Sprouts
Broccoli Florets
Broccoli Spears
Cauliflower Florets
Cabbage
Courgettes
Cut Leeks
Diced Swede
Sliced Onions
Leaf Spinach
Baked Potato Halves
Baked Potato Halves with
    Cheese & Ham
Baked Potato Halves with
    Chicken & Sweetcorn

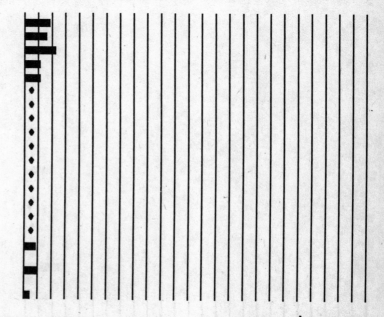

♦ = negligible

Grams per 25g/1oz (approx)

Item	1	2	3	4	5	6	7	8	9	10	11	12	13	14	15	16	17	18	19	20	21	22	23	24	25
Baked Potato Halves with Garlic Butter	██																								
Sweetcorn	█																								
Button Mushrooms	███																								
Sliced Mushrooms	◆																								
Petits Champignons	◆																								
Mixed Peppers	◆																								
Parsnips	◆																								
Broccoli Mix	◆																								
Sweetcorn & Pepper Mix	█																								
Crispy Coated Onion Rings	███																								
Mixed Melon Balls	◆																								
Carrot & Swede Mix	◆																								
Chinese Mix	◆																								
Hawaiian Mix	◆																								
Julienne Mix	◆																								
Country Style Vegetable Mix	◆																								
Indian Pilau Rice	█																								
Mixed Vegetables	◆																								

Stewpack

NESTLE (Findus)
Asparagus Spears
Beans – Sliced Green
Broad Beans
Broccoli Spears
Brussel Sprouts
Cauliflower Fleurettes
Corn on the Cob
Country Mix Vegetables
Haricot Verts
Peas
Petit Pois
Mange Tout
Minted Peas
Mixed Vegetables
Spinach – Chopped
Spinach – Creamed
Spinach – Mornay
Spinach – Whole Leaf

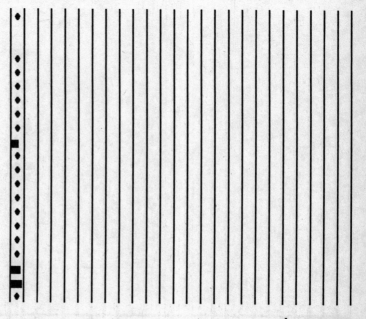

♦ = negligible

Grams per 25g/1oz (approx)	1	2	3	4	5	6	7	8	9	10	11	12	13	14	15	16	17	18	19	20	21	22	23	24	25
Sweetcorn Kernels	■																								
Crinkle Cut Chips	■																								
3-Way Cook Chips	■																								
Saute Potatoes	■																								
Crinkle-Cut Jackets	■																								

SAINSBURYS

Frozen

	1	2	3	4	5	6	7	8	9	10	11	12	13	14	15	16	17	18	19	20	21	22	23	24	25
Ovenbaked Parsnips	■																								
Broad Beans	◆																								
Cut Beans	◆																								
Sliced Beans	◆																								
Whole Beans	◆																								
Broccoli Spears	◆																								
Cabbage - Sliced	◆																								
Baby Carrots	◆																								
Cauliflower Florets	◆																								
Hash Browns - Shallow Fried	■																								

411

Oven Jacket Scallops - Oven Baked	
Mixed Vegetables	
Button Mushrooms - Fried	
Crispy Coated Mushrooms	
Economy Peas	
Garden Peas	
Minted Peas	
Petit Pois	
Potato Bake	
Crinkle Cut Potato Chips - Deep Fried	
Oven Potato Chips - Oven Baked	
Steak Potato Chips - Deep Fried	
Straight Cut Potato Chips - Deep Fried	
Potato Waffles - Shallow Fried	
Ovensteak Potatoes	

♦ = negligible

Grams per 25g/1oz (approx)	1	2	3	4	5	6	7	8	9	10	11	12	13	14	15	16	17	18	19	20	21	22	23	24	25
American Style Fries – Fried	███																								
Chopped Spinach	◆																								
Sprouts	◆																								
Button Sprouts	◆																								
Stew Pack	◆																								
Diced Swede – Boiled	◆																								
Sweetcorn	█																								
Sweetcorn & Peppers	█																								
Salad Vegetables																									
Bean Sprouts	◆																								
Celery	◆																								
Chicory	◆																								
Chinese Leaf	◆																								
Cucumber	◆																								
Cos Lettuce	◆																								
Feuille de Chene Lettuce	◆																								
Iceberg Lettuce	◆																								
Little Gem Lettuce	◆																								

Lollo Rosso Lettuce ♦
Round Lettuce ♦
Quattro Stagioni Lettuce ♦
Radish ♦
Cherry Tomatoes ♦
Round Tomatoes ♦
Watercress ♦

Other
Artichoke - Globe ♦
Asparagus ♦
Aubergine ♦
Beetroot ♦
Broad Beans - Boiled ♦
Broccoli Tops ♦
Brussels Sprouts ♦
Cabbage - Red ♦
Cabbage - Savoy ♦
Cabbage - White ♦
Carrots - Boiled ♦
Cauliflower ♦

♦ = negligible

Grams per 25g/1oz (approx)	1	2	3	4	5	6	7	8	9	10	11	12	13	14	15	16	17	18	19	20	21	22	23	24	25
Courgettes – Raw	●																								
Eddoes – Raw	●																								
Fennel – Boiled	‖																								
Garlic – Boiled	●																								
Ginger Root – Raw	‖																								
Karela	●																								
Kohl Rabi	●																								
Leeks – Boiled	●																								
Mangetout	●																								
Marrow	●																								
Matoki	●																								
Mooli – Boiled	●																								
Mushrooms Button – Raw	●																								
Mushrooms Large Flat – Raw	●																								
Okra	●																								
Onions	●																								
Parsnips – Boiled	‖																								
Peanuts – Roasted	███████████████████████																								
Peas – Boiled	●																								

415

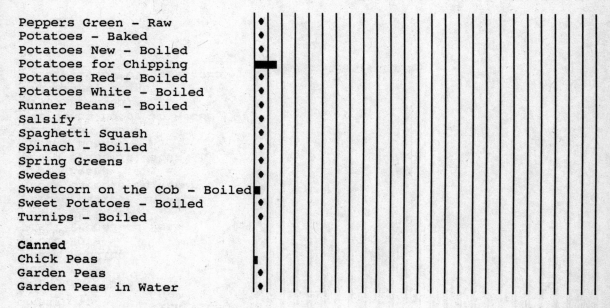

```
Peppers Green - Raw             ◆
Potatoes - Baked                ◆
Potatoes New - Boiled           ◆
Potatoes for Chipping           ▬▬
Potatoes Red - Boiled           ◆
Potatoes White - Boiled         ◆
Runner Beans - Boiled           ◆
Salsify                         ◆
Spaghetti Squash                ◆
Spinach - Boiled                ◆
Spring Greens                   ◆
Swedes                          ◆
Sweetcorn on the Cob - Boiled   ▪
Sweet Potatoes - Boiled         ◆
Turnips - Boiled                ◆

Canned
Chick Peas                      ▪
Garden Peas                     ◆
Garden Peas in Water            ◆
```

◆ = negligible

Grams per 25g/1oz (approx)	1	2	3	4	5	6	7	8	9	10	11	12	13	14	15	16	17	18	19	20	21	22	23	24	25
Marrow Fat Peas with Vinegar & Mint	•																								
Marrowfat Peas	•																								
Mushy Peas	•																								
Pease Pudding	•																								
Petit Pois	•																								
Small Processed Peas	•																								
Young Carrots	•																								
Sliced Carrots in Water	•																								
Whole Carrots in Water	•																								
Broad Beans	•																								
Broad Beans in Water	•																								
Chilli Beans	‖																								
Cut Green Beans	•																								
Cut Green Beans in Water	•																								
Mixed Bean Salad	‖																								
Red Kidney Beans	•																								
Naturally Sweet Sweetcorn	■																								

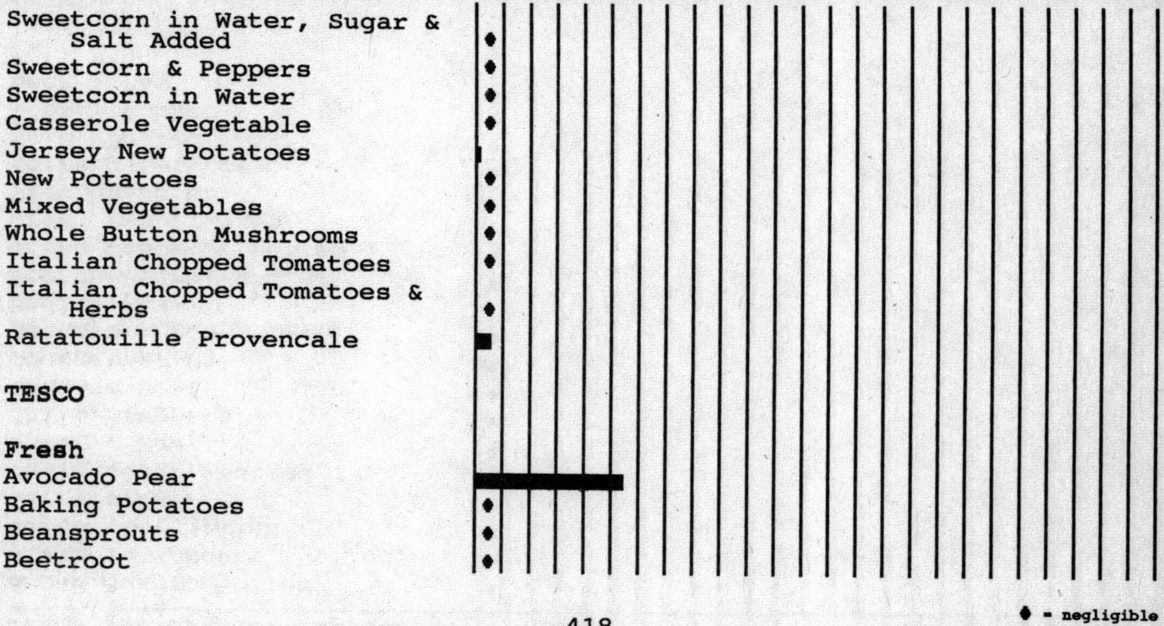

Sweetcorn in Water, Sugar & Salt Added	♦
Sweetcorn & Peppers	♦
Sweetcorn in Water	♦
Casserole Vegetable	♦
Jersey New Potatoes	▌
New Potatoes	♦
Mixed Vegetables	♦
Whole Button Mushrooms	♦
Italian Chopped Tomatoes	♦
Italian Chopped Tomatoes & Herbs	♦
Ratatouille Provencale	■

TESCO

Fresh

Avocado Pear	▬▬▬▬▬
Baking Potatoes	♦
Beansprouts	♦
Beetroot	♦

♦ = negligible

Grams per 25g/1oz (approx)	1	2	3	4	5	6	7	8	9	10	11	12	13	14	15	16	17	18	19	20	21	22	23	24	25
Broad Beans, Boiled	•																								
Brussels Sprouts, Boiled	•																								
Calabrese, Boiled	•																								
Carrots, Raw	•																								
Cauliflower, Boiled	•																								
Celery, Raw	•																								
Chilli Peppers	•																								
Chinese Leaf	•																								
Courgette, Raw	•																								
Cucumber, Raw	•																								
Endive, Raw	•																								
French Beans, Cooked	•																								
Green Cabbage, Boiled	•																								
Green Pepper, Raw	•																								
Growing Salad																									
Iceberg Lettuce	•																								
Kale, Boiled	•																								
Leeks, Cooked	•																								
Leeks, Raw	•																								

Lettuce, Round/Cos/Crisp	♦
Marrow, Boiled	♦
Mushrooms, Fried	▬▬▬▬▬▬
Mushrooms, Raw	♦
Mustard & Cress	♦
New Potatoes, Boiled	♦
Onions, Boiled	♦
Onions, Fried	▬▬▬▬▬▬▬▬
Parsley	♦
Parsnips, Boiled	♦
Peas, Cooked	♦
Peas, Raw	♦
Potatoes (Old), Boiled	♦
Pumpkin, Boiled	♦
Radishes	♦
Red Cabbage, Raw	♦
Red Pepper	♦
Red Radish, Cooked	▮
Salsify, Cooked	♦
Shallot, Raw	♦
Spinach, Boiled	♦

♦ = negligible

Grams per 25g/1oz (approx)	1	2	3	4	5	6	7	8	9	10	11	12	13	14	15	16	17	18	19	20	21	22	23	24	25
Spring Greens, Boiled	◆																								
Spring Onions	◆																								
Squash (Spaghetti)	◆																								
Squash (Winter)	◆																								
Swede, Cooked	◆																								
Swede, Raw	◆																								
Sweetcorn on Cob, Boiled	■																								
Tomatoes, Raw	◆																								
Turnips, Boiled	◆																								
Watercress	◆																								
White Cabbage, Raw	◆																								
Yellow Pepper	◆																								
Exotic																									
Asparagus, Cooked	◆																								
Aubergine, Raw	◆																								
Bobby Beans, Cooked	▮																								
Celeriac, Cooked	◆																								
Chicory, Cooked	◆																								

421

```
Chicory, Raw              ♦
Eddoes, Cooked            ▌
Eddoes, Raw               ♦
Fennel, Cooked            ▌
Fennel, Raw               ♦
Fine Beans, Cooked        ♦
Fine Beans, Raw           ♦
Garlic, Raw               ♦
Ginger Root, Raw          ▌
Globe Artichoke, Cooked   ♦
Jerusalem Artichoke, Cooked ♦
Kohl Rabi, Raw            ♦
Mange Tout, Cooked        ♦
Mange Tout, Raw           ♦
Mooli, Raw                ♦
Okra, Raw                 ♦
Sweet Potato, Cooked      ♦
Sweet Potato, Raw         ♦
Yam, Cooked               ♦
Yam, Raw                  ♦
```

♦ = negligible

Grams per 25g/1oz (approx)	1	2	3	4	5	6	7	8	9	10	11	12	13	14	15	16	17	18	19	20	21	22	23	24	25
Dried																									
Instant Mashed Potato (made up)	♦																								
Mixed Pepper	▬																								
Mixed Vegetables	♦																								
Mushroom Slices	♦																								
Peas, Cooked	♦																								
Sliced Onions	♦																								
Canned																									
Broad Beans	♦																								
Butter Beans	♦																								
Carrots – No Added Salt	♦																								
Chopped Tomatoes	♦																								
Creamed Mushrooms	▬																								
Crinkle Cut Carrots	♦																								
Cut Green Beans	♦																								
Economy Potatoes	♦																								
Garden Peas	♦																								

Garden Peas - No Added Sugar/Salt	♦
Jersey New Potatoes	♦
Mixed Vegetables	♦
New Potatoes	♦
Petit Pois	♦
Plum Tomatoes	♦
Processed Marrowfat Peas	♦
Processed Peas	♦
Ratatouille	▮
Sliced Button Mushrooms	♦
Sliced Carrots	♦
Sliced Green Beans	♦
Sliced Large Mushrooms	♦
Summer Mixed Vegetables	♦
Sweetcorn with Peppers	♦
Sweetcorn	♦
Unpeeled Jersey New Potatoes	♦
Whole Baby Carrots	♦
Whole Button Mushrooms	▮
Whole Carrots	♦

♦ = negligible

Grams per 25g/1oz (approx)	1	2	3	4	5	6	7	8	9	10	11	12	13	14	15	16	17	18	19	20	21	22	23	24	25
Whole Green Beans	♦																								
Frozen																									
Broccoli Spears	♦																								
Brown Rice with Mixed Vegetables	♦																								
Brussels Sprouts	♦																								
Broad Beans	♦																								
Cabbage	♦																								
Carrots	♦																								
Casserole Mixed Vegetables	♦																								
Cauliflower Florets	♦																								
Corn-on-the-Cob	■																								
Farmhouse Mixed Vegetables	♦																								
Green Beans	♦																								
Leaf Spinach	♦																								
Manor Mixed Vegetables	♦																								
Mini Corn-on-the-Cob	■																								
Mixed Peppers	♦																								

Mixed Vegetables	◆
Mushrooms	◆
Onions (Fried)	
Oven Chips	
Parisienne Carrots	◆
Parisienne Mixed Vegetables	
Ratatouille Mixed Vegetables	
Sliced Courgettes	◆
Special Mixed Vegetables	
Steakhouse Chips	
Straight Cut Chips	
Straight Cut Oven Chips	
Sweetcorn Kernels	

Jars

Baby Carrots	◆
Broad Beans	◆
Cut Green Beans	◆
Peas & Carrots	◆

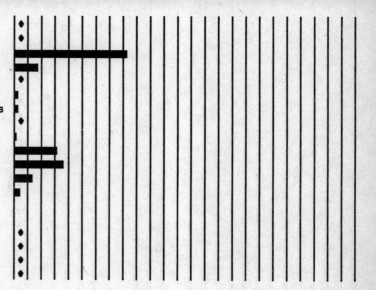

426

◆ = negligible

Grams per 25g/1oz (approx)	1	2	3	4	5	6	7	8	9	10	11	12	13	14	15	16	17	18	19	20	21	22	23	24	25
Stir Fries																									
Chinese Style	◆																								
Country Style	◆																								
Eastern Style	◆																								
Indian Style	■																								
WAITROSE																									
Fresh																									
Beetroot Cooked	◆																								
Beetroot Uncooked	◆																								
Broccoli	◆																								
Brussels Sprouts	◆																								
Carrots	◆																								
Cauliflower	◆																								
Celery	◆																								
Chicory	◆																								
Courgettes	◆																								
Cucumber	◆																								

427

Finger Carrots	◆
Globe Artichokes	◆
Green Peppers	◆
Jerusalem Artichokes	◆
Leeks	◆
Lettuce	◆
Mooli	◆
Mushrooms	◆
Onions	◆
Parsley	◆
Parsnips	◆
Peas	◆
Potatoes	◆
Pumpkin	◆
Red Cabbage	◆
Shallots	◆
Spinach	◆
Sprouting Broccoli	◆
Swedes	◆
Sweetcorn	■
Tomatoes	◆

◆ = negligible

Grams per 25g/1oz (approx)	1	2	3	4	5	6	7	8	9	10	11	12	13	14	15	16	17	18	19	20	21	22	23	24	25
Turnips	♦																								
White Cabbage	♦																								
Frozen																									
Broad Beans	♦																								
Sliced Green Beans	♦																								
Whole Green Beans	♦																								
Cauliflower, Broccoli & Carrots	♦																								
Cauliflower Florets	♦																								
Corn Cobs	■																								
Mini Corn Cobs	▌																								
Garden Peas	♦																								
Mint Peas	♦																								
Peas	♦																								
Peas, Corn & Pepper	▌																								
Petit Pois	♦																								
Sprouts	♦																								
Leaf Spinach	♦																								

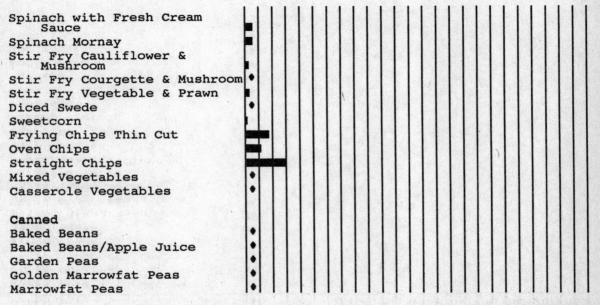

Spinach with Fresh Cream Sauce	
Spinach Mornay	
Stir Fry Cauliflower & Mushroom	
Stir Fry Courgette & Mushroom	♦
Stir Fry Vegetable & Prawn	
Diced Swede	♦
Sweetcorn	
Frying Chips Thin Cut	
Oven Chips	
Straight Chips	
Mixed Vegetables	♦
Casserole Vegetables	♦
Canned	
Baked Beans	♦
Baked Beans/Apple Juice	♦
Garden Peas	♦
Golden Marrowfat Peas	♦
Marrowfat Peas	♦

♦ = negligible

430

Grams per 25g/1oz (approx)	1	2	3	4	5	6	7	8	9	10	11	12	13	14	15	16	17	18	19	20	21	22	23	24	25
Petit Pois	♦																								
Petit Pois with Carrots	♦																								
Processed Peas	♦																								
Small Processed Peas	♦																								
Broad Beans	♦																								
Kidney Beans	♦																								
Chick Peas	▌																								
Cut Green Beans	♦																								
Whole Green Beans	♦																								
Haricots Verts	♦																								
Butter Beans	♦																								
Baby Carrots	♦																								
Carrots	♦																								
Sliced Carrots	♦																								
Tomatoes	♦																								
Crushed Tomatoes	♦																								
Passata	♦																								
Potatoes	♦																								
New Potatoes	♦																								

431

Jersey Potatoes	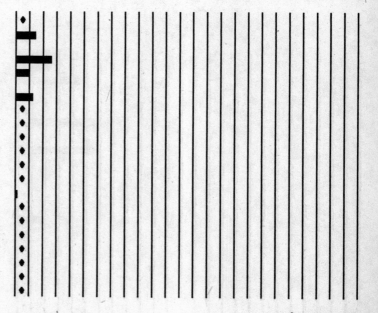
Potato Fry	
Saute Potato Egg, Bacon & Onion	
Saute Potato Onion & Bacon	
Saute Potato Onion, Sausage & Cheese	
Artichokes	
Asparagus Cuts/tips	
Asparagus Spears	
Canadian Green Asparagus	
Celery Hearts	
Cream Style Corn	
Sweetcorn	
Sweetcorn with Peppers	
Sweetcorn - No Added Sugar	
Sweet Red Peppers	
Spinach	
Button Mushrooms	
Chopped Mushrooms	
Macedoine of Veg	

♦ = negligible

432

Grams per 25g/1oz (approx)	1	2	3	4	5	6	7	8	9	10	11	12	13	14	15	16	17	18	19	20	21	22	23	24	25
Mixed Vegetables																									
Ratatouille																									

VEGETARIAN FOODS

DIETBURGER COMPANY LIMITED
Dietburger																									

BOOTS
Soup:
Bean & Pepper																									
Country Mushroom																									
Country Vegetable																									
Farm Celery																									
Potato & Leek																									
Red Lentil																									
Savoury Tomato																									
Spring Vegetable																									
Spicy Vegetable Soup																									

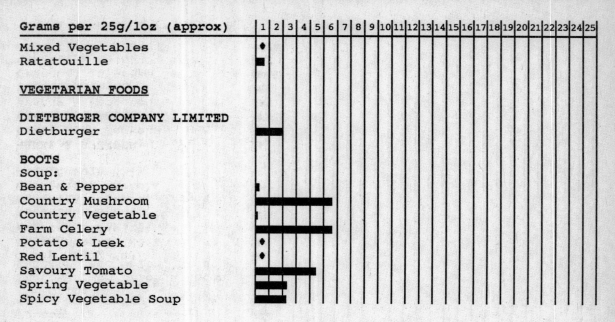

Vegetarian Green Bean Soup
Vegetarian Thick Lentil Soup
Vegetarian Thick Potato Soup
Aubergine Moussaka Ready Meal
Country Casserole Ready Meal
Curry Ready Meal
Lasagne Ready Meal
Vegetable Masala Ready Meal
Macaroni Cheese Medley
Tagliatelle Verdi
Wholewheat Ravioli
Liquid Soya Milk

MARKS & SPENCER
Baked Bean Jackets
Baked Potato with Cheese
Brandy & Peppercorn Sauce
Bread Sauce
Broccoli in Cream Sauce
Cabbage & Mushroom Bake
Cauliflower Cheese

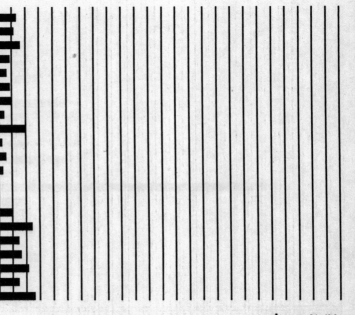

◆ = negligible

Grams per 25g/1oz (approx)

Food	Grams (approx)
Chasseur Sauce	1
Cheese & Mushroom Sauce	2
Chinese Style Rice	1
Cocktail Spring Rolls	3
Creamy Potato Gratin	2
Crispy Mushrooms	3
Filled Green Pepper	1
Fresh Vegetable Bake	2
Fresh Vegetable Dip	20
Garden Vegetable Pie	2
Garlic Mushrooms	4
Kiev Jacket Potato	2
Leek & Carrot Jacket Potato	2
Mushroom Jacket Potato	2
Onion Bhajjis	5
Pancakes, Mushroom in Beer Batter	3
Potato Bake	2
Potato Croquettes	1

Ratatouille
Red Cabbage with Apple
Vegetable Lasagne
Vegetable Chilli
Vegetable Cutlets
Vegetable Samosa

NESTLE (Findus - Natural
Choice)
Broccoli in Cheese Sauce
Cauliflower Cheese
Cheese Cannelloni
Green Bean & Mushroom Bake

SAINSBURYS
Broccoli Provencale
Cauliflower Cheese
Courgette Provencale
Lasagne Pomodoro
Mushroom & Ricotta Cheese
Cannelloni

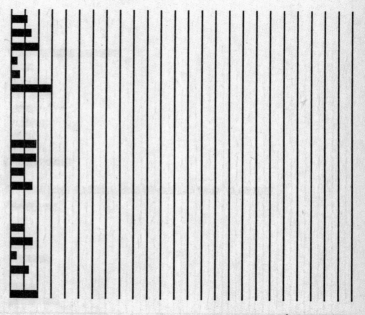

♦ = negligible

Grams per 25g/1oz (approx)

Food	Grams per 25g/1oz (approx)
Onion Bhajia	4
Potato Dauphinoise	2
Potato, Leek & Celery Bake	1
Sate & Peanut Sauce Dip	4
Vegetable Mornay	2
Vegetable Chilli with Cracked Wheat	2
Vegetable Samosas	4
TESCO	
Broccoli Mornay	2
Cabbage & Mushroom Bake	2
Carrot & Onion Crumble	3
Cauliflower Cheese	3
Cheesy Potato Bake	2
Country Vegetable Quiche	4
Leek & Potato Bake	1
Vegetable Bake	2
Vegetarian Cheddar Cheese	9

437

Vegetable Curry
Vegetable Flan
Vegetable Lasagne
Vegetable Moussaka
Vegetarian Red Leicester
    Cheese

WAITROSE
Aubergine Gratin
Agnolotti Vegetariani –
    Cooked
Broccoli & Swiss Cheese
    Quiche
Cauliflower Cheese
Potato Dauphinoise
Ratatouille
Vegetable Shepherds Pie
Vegetable Chilli
Vegetable Stroganoff
Vegetable Casserole
Vegetable Moussaka

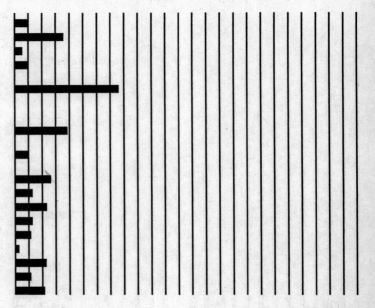

♦ = negligible

438

Grams per 25g/1oz (approx)	1	2	3	4	5	6	7	8	9	10	11	12	13	14	15	16	17	18	19	20	21	22	23	24	25
Vegetable Burrito																									
Vegetable Lasagne																									
Vegetable Samosa																									

YOGURT & DESSERTS - GENERAL

Yogurt (low fat)

	1	2	3	4	5	6	7	8	9	10	11	12	13	14	15	16	17	18	19	20	21	22	23	24	25
Diet (all flavours)																									
Natural																									
Flavoured																									
Fruit																									
Hazelnut																									
Diet French Style Set Yogurt																									
Strained Greek Ewes																									

BOOTS

	1	2	3	4	5	6	7	8	9	10	11	12	13	14	15	16	17	18	19	20	21	22	23	24	25
Dessert - Gooseberry Cream																									
Dessert - Rhubarb Cream																									
Dessert - Strawberry Cream																									

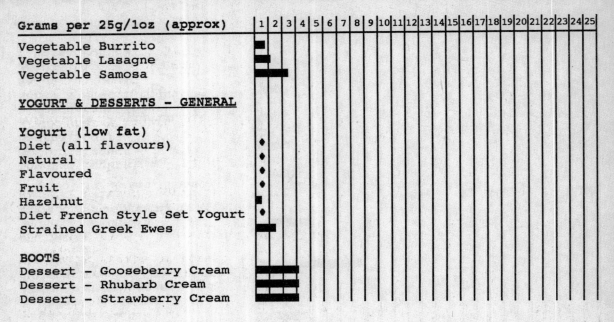

Shapers Citrus Fruit Dessert

Shapers English Garden Fruit
    Dessert

Shapers Strawberry Dessert

Shapers Tropical Dessert

Wholemilk Fruits of Forest
    Yogurt

Wholemilk Plum & Apple Yogurt

BRIDGE FARM DAIRIES LIMITED
Natural Stirred Yogurt

Low Fat Yogurt:
Apricot Yogurt

Banana Yogurt

Black Cherry Yogurt

Blackcurrant Yogurt

Honey & Muesli Yogurt

Mandarin Yogurt

Natural Stirred Yogurt

Natural Pot Set Yogurt

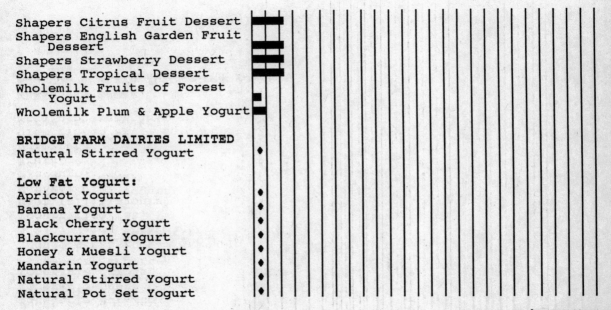

♦ = negligible

Grams per 25g/1oz (approx)	1	2	3	4	5	6	7	8	9	10	11	12	13	14	15	16	17	18	19	20	21	22	23	24	25
Peach Melba Yogurt	◆																								
Pineapple Yogurt	◆																								
Raspberry Yogurt	◆																								
Strawberry Yogurt	◆																								
Very Low Fat Pasteurized Yogurt:																									
Apricot Yogurt	◆																								
Black Cherry Yogurt	◆																								
Mandarin Yogurt	◆																								
Natural Yogurt	◆																								
Peach Yogurt	◆																								
Raspberry Yogurt	◆																								
Strawberry Yogurt	◆																								
MARKS & SPENCER																									
Apricot & Guava Thick Creamy Yogurt	■																								

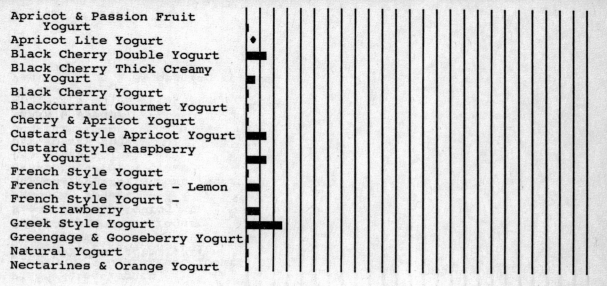

Apricot & Passion Fruit Yogurt	
Apricot Lite Yogurt	♦
Black Cherry Double Yogurt	
Black Cherry Thick Creamy Yogurt	
Black Cherry Yogurt	
Blackcurrant Gourmet Yogurt	
Cherry & Apricot Yogurt	
Custard Style Apricot Yogurt	
Custard Style Raspberry Yogurt	
French Style Yogurt	
French Style Yogurt – Lemon	
French Style Yogurt – Strawberry	
Greek Style Yogurt	
Greengage & Gooseberry Yogurt	
Natural Yogurt	
Nectarines & Orange Yogurt	

♦ = negligible

Grams per 25g/1oz (approx)	1	2	3	4	5	6	7	8	9	10	11	12	13	14	15	16	17	18	19	20	21	22	23	24	25
Orange Thick and Creamy Yogurt	■																								
Peach Melba Yogurt	▌																								
Pineapple & Grapefruit Yogurt	▎																								
Raspberry & Passion Fruit Yogurt	■																								
Raspberry Gourmet Yogurt	▎																								
Raspberry Ripple Yogurt	■																								
Rhubarb Yogurt	▎																								
Strawberry & Wild Herb Yogurt	■																								
Strawberry Thick Creamy Yogurt	■																								
Strawberry Yogurt	▌																								
Sunfruit Yogurt	▎																								
Thick & Creamy Fruits of Forest	■																								
Toffee Yogurt	▎																								
Vanilla Rich & Smooth Yogurt	██																								

443

Whole Milk French Yogurt –
   Natural

NESTLE (Chambourcy)

Bonjour Yogurts – Set
Fruit Flavour Varieties
Natural

Nouvelle Yogurts
Apricot & Apple
Black Cherry
Hazelnut & Apple
Hippo Low Fat Set with
   Vitamins A,C,D
Peach & Passion Fruit
Peach & Redcurrant
Pear & Banana
Raspberry
Raspberry & Kumquat
Strawberry

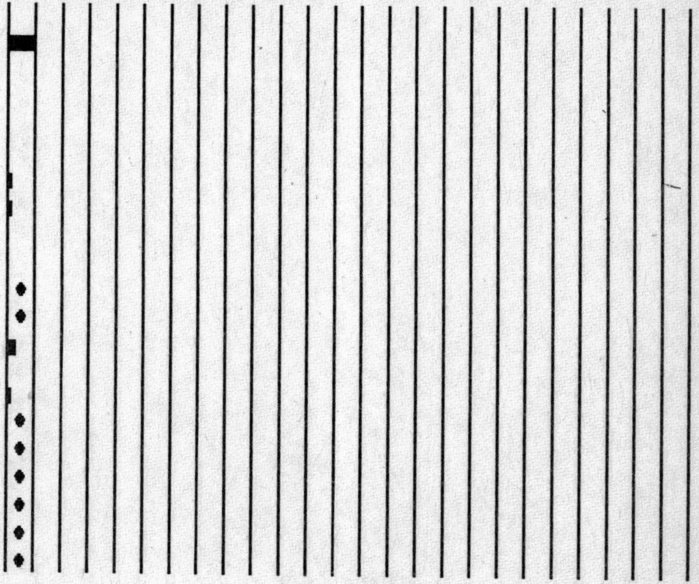

444

♦ = negligible

Grams per 25g/1oz (approx)	1	2	3	4	5	6	7	8	9	10	11	12	13	14	15	16	17	18	19	20	21	22	23	24	25
Strawberry & Lychee	♦																								
Strawberry Plus Flavours	♦																								
Walnut & Melon	▮																								
Robot Yogurts																									
Banana	♦																								
Black Cherry	♦																								
Pot au Chocolate	▬																								
Pot au Creme	▬																								
Raspberry	♦																								
Strawberry	♦																								
SAINSBURYS																									
Black Cherry Diet Yogurt	♦																								
Fruits of Forest Diet Yogurt	♦																								
Nectarine & Apricot Diet Yogurt	♦																								
Rhubarb Diet Yogurt	♦																								
Strawberry Diet Yogurt	♦																								

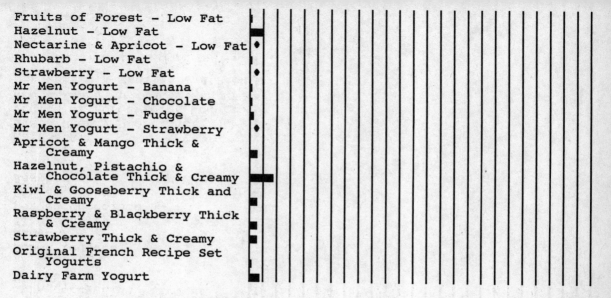

Fruits of Forest – Low Fat	
Hazelnut – Low Fat	
Nectarine & Apricot – Low Fat	◆
Rhubarb – Low Fat	
Strawberry – Low Fat	◆
Mr Men Yogurt – Banana	
Mr Men Yogurt – Chocolate	
Mr Men Yogurt – Fudge	
Mr Men Yogurt – Strawberry	◆
Apricot & Mango Thick & Creamy	
Hazelnut, Pistachio & Chocolate Thick & Creamy	
Kiwi & Gooseberry Thick and Creamy	
Raspberry & Blackberry Thick & Creamy	
Strawberry Thick & Creamy	
Original French Recipe Set Yogurts	
Dairy Farm Yogurt	

446

◆ = negligible

Grams per 25g/1oz (approx)	1	2	3	4	5	6	7	8	9	10	11	12	13	14	15	16	17	18	19	20	21	22	23	24	25
Exotic French Recipe Yogurts	▮																								
Natural Yogurt	▮																								
ST IVEL																									
Shape Yogurt																									
Black Cherry	♦																								
Muesli	♦																								
Natural	♦																								
Peach Melba	♦																								
Raspberry	♦																								
Rhubarb	♦																								
Strawberry	♦																								
Fruits of Forest – 4 Pack	♦																								
Passion Fruit & Melon – 4 Pack	♦																								
Strawberry & Vanilla – 4 Pack	♦																								

447

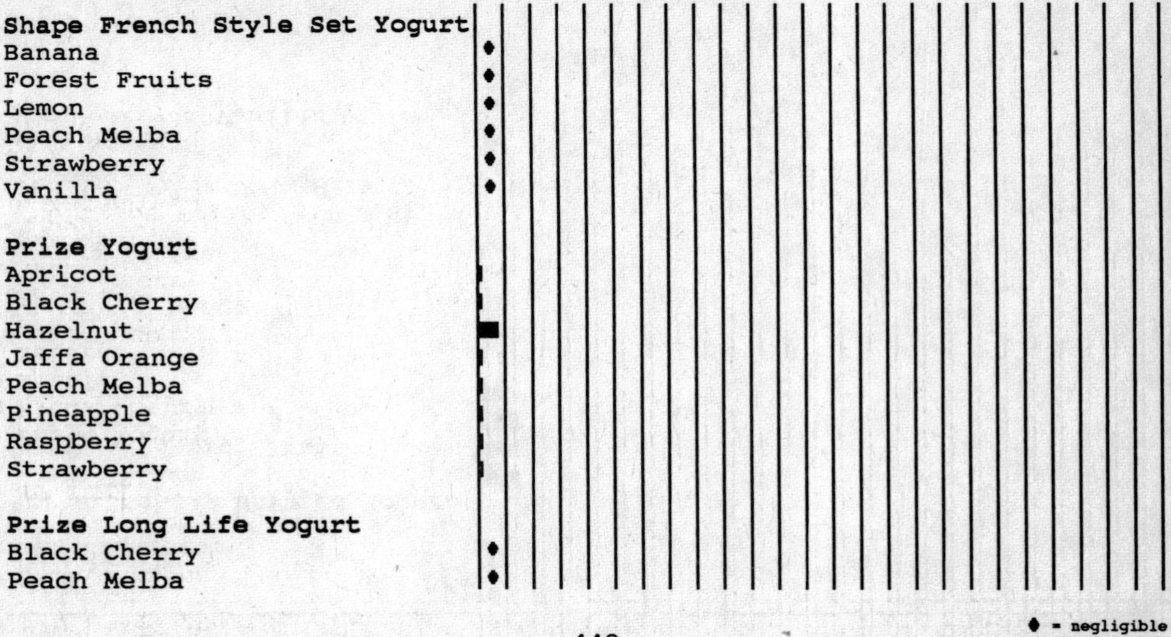

Shape French Style Set Yogurt
Banana
Forest Fruits
Lemon
Peach Melba
Strawberry
Vanilla

Prize Yogurt
Apricot
Black Cherry
Hazelnut
Jaffa Orange
Peach Melba
Pineapple
Raspberry
Strawberry

Prize Long Life Yogurt
Black Cherry
Peach Melba

♦ = negligible

Grams per 25g/1oz (approx)	1	2	3	4	5	6	7	8	9	10	11	12	13	14	15	16	17	18	19	20	21	22	23	24	25
Raspberry	•																								
Strawberry	•																								
Prize Lightly Whipped Yogurt																									
Lemon & Lime	■																								
Peach & Passion Fruit	■																								
Raspberry	■																								
Strawberry	■																								
Real Yogurt																									
Apricot & Mango	▮																								
Black Cherry	▮																								
Forest Fruits	▮																								
Orange	▮																								
Peach Melba	▮																								
Raspberry	▮																								
Real Active	■																								
Strawberry & Vanilla	▮																								

TESCO
Apple & Cinnamon
Apple & Mango
Apricot
Apricot & Mango
Banana
Banana Surprise
Blackcherry
Blackberry and Apple
Blackcurrant
Boysenberry & Apple
Breakfast Bowl - Apple
Breakfast Bowl - Orange
Cherry & Almond
Chocolate
Coconut
French Set - All Flavours
Fruits of the Forest
Gooseberry
Greek Style
Hazelnut

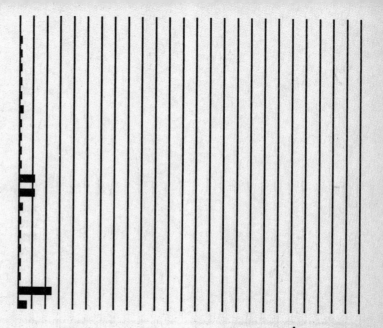

450

♦ = negligible

Grams per 25g/1oz (approx)	1	2	3	4	5	6	7	8	9	10	11	12	13	14	15	16	17	18	19	20	21	22	23	24	25
Mandarin & Grapefruit																									
Mango & Lime																									
Natural																									
Natural Set																									
Nectarine & Apricot																									
Orange																									
Orange & Watermelon																									
Passion Fruit and Melon																									
Peach																									
Peach Melba																									
Pineapple																									
Plum																									
Raspberry																									
Real French Set																									
Rhubarb																									
Rich & Creamy French Set – All Flavours																									
Strawberry																									
Strawberry & Lychee																									

Strawberry & Mango
Strawberry & Peach
Strawberry & Vanilla
Toffee
Tropical Fruit
Very Low Fat Yogurt - All
    Flavours
Whipping Yogurt

American Style:
Banana & Butterscotch
Blueberry
Chocolate Fudge
Orange Cream Soda

Childrens Range:
Banana
Blackcurrant
Chocolate
Fudge
Raspberry

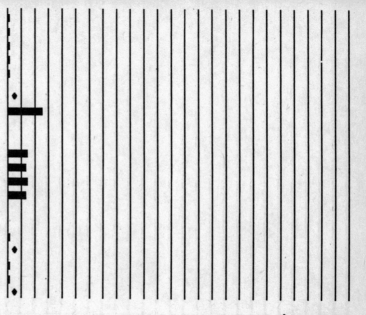

◆ = negligible

Grams per 25g/1oz (approx)	1	2	3	4	5	6	7	8	9	10	11	12	13	14	15	16	17	18	19	20	21	22	23	24	25
Strawberry																									
Toffee	♦																								
Healthy Eating:																									
Apricot & Mango	♦																								
Banana	♦																								
Black Cherry	♦																								
Mandarin	♦																								
Melon	♦																								
Natural	♦																								
Peach Melba	♦																								
Pineapple	♦																								
Raspberry	♦																								
Rhubarb	♦																								
Strawberry	♦																								
Longlife:																									
Banana	♦																								
Black Cherry	♦																								

Mandarin
Peach Melba
Raspberry
Rhubarb
Strawberry
Toffee Apple

Reduced Sugar:
Black Cherry
Peach Melba
Raspberry
Strawberry

Thick & Creamy:
Black Cherry
Coffee & Walnut
Forest Fruit
Mango & Apricot
Orange & Chocolate
Peach & Kumquat
Raspberry & Passion Fruit

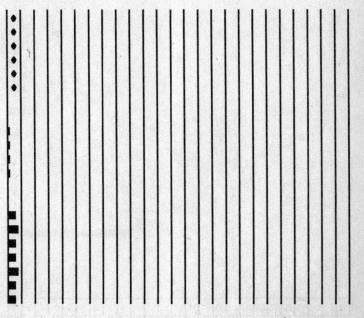

♦ = negligible

Grams per 25g/1oz (approx)	1	2	3	4	5	6	7	8	9	10	11	12	13	14	15	16	17	18	19	20	21	22	23	24	25
Strawberry																									
Strawberry & Vanilla																									
Toffee 7 Nut																									
WAITROSE																									
Yogurt Dressing																									
Apricot Yogurt																									
Banana Yogurt																									
Black Cherry Yogurt																									
Blackberry & Apple Yogurt																									
Blackcurrant Yogurt																									
Champ Rhubarb Yogurt																									
Chocolate Yogurt																									
Creamy Blackcurrant & Rosehip Yogurt																									
Creamy Fruits of Forest Yogurt																									
Creamy Raspberry & Melon Yogurt																									

Creamy Strawberry Yogurt	
Diet Yogurt	
French Light Set Yogurt	
Fruits of Forest Yogurt	
Gooseberry Yogurt	
Hazelnut Yogurt	
Low Fat Yogurt	
Mandarin Yogurt	
Natural Yogurt	
Natural Set Yogurt	
Passion Fruit & Melon Yogurt	
Peach Melba Yogurt	
Raspberry Yogurt	
Strawberry Yogurt	
Victoria Plum Yogurt	

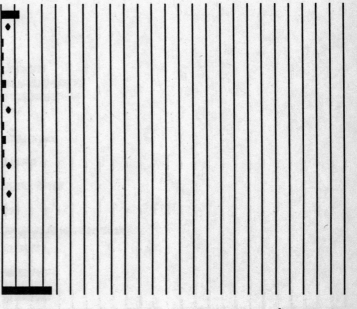

EATING OUT

BOOTS
Bacon, Lettuce & Tomato
    Sandwich

◆ = negligible

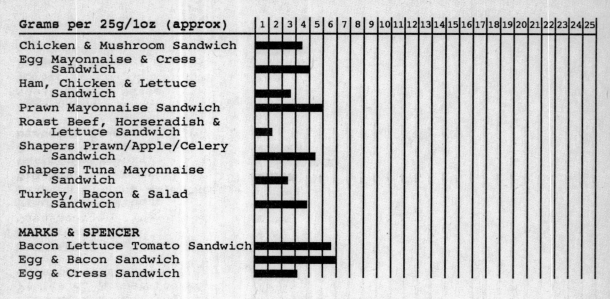

Grams per 25g/1oz (approx)	1	2	3	4	5	6	7	8	9	10	11	12	13	14	15	16	17	18	19	20	21	22	23	24	25
Chicken & Mushroom Sandwich																									
Egg Mayonnaise & Cress Sandwich																									
Ham, Chicken & Lettuce Sandwich																									
Prawn Mayonnaise Sandwich																									
Roast Beef, Horseradish & Lettuce Sandwich																									
Shapers Prawn/Apple/Celery Sandwich																									
Shapers Tuna Mayonnaise Sandwich																									
Turkey, Bacon & Salad Sandwich																									
MARKS & SPENCER																									
Bacon Lettuce Tomato Sandwich																									
Egg & Bacon Sandwich																									
Egg & Cress Sandwich																									

Prawn & Mayonnaise Sandwich
Roast Chicken & Salad
       Sandwich
Salmon & Cucumber Sandwich
Turkey & Ham Sandwich

McDONALD'S
Hamburger
Cheeseburger
Quarter Pounder
Quarter Pounder with Cheese
Big Mac
Fillet-O-Fish
Chicken McNuggets
Barbecue Sauce
Sweet Curry Sauce
Mild Mustard Sauce
Sweet & Sour Sauce
Tomato Ketchup Portion
French Fries
Apple Pie

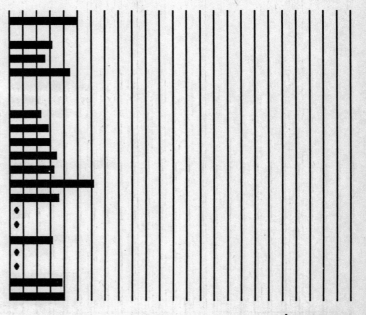

◆ = negligible

Grams per 25g/1oz (approx)

Item	Grams per 25g/1oz (approx)
Vanilla Flavour Milkshake	1
Strawberry Flavour Milkshake	1
Chocolate Flavour Milkshake	1
McDonald's Cola	•
Diet McDonald's Cola	•
McDonald's Orange Drink	•
McDonald's Root Beer	•
Milk	
White Coffee	2
Scrambled Eggs	2½
Sausage Pattie	8
English Muffin with Butter	2
English Muffin with Butter & Jam	2
Hash Brown Potato	5
Bacon & Egg Muffin	2
Sausage & Egg Muffin	5
Hotcakes with Butter & Syrup	1
Apple Danish	4

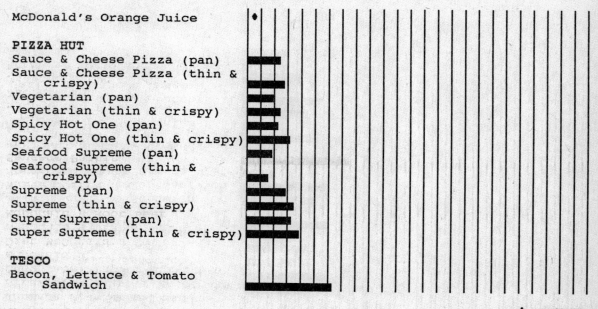

McDonald's Orange Juice

PIZZA HUT
Sauce & Cheese Pizza (pan)
Sauce & Cheese Pizza (thin & crispy)
Vegetarian (pan)
Vegetarian (thin & crispy)
Spicy Hot One (pan)
Spicy Hot One (thin & crispy)
Seafood Supreme (pan)
Seafood Supreme (thin & crispy)
Supreme (pan)
Supreme (thin & crispy)
Super Supreme (pan)
Super Supreme (thin & crispy)

TESCO
Bacon, Lettuce & Tomato Sandwich

460

♦ = negligible

Grams per 25g/1oz (approx)	1	2	3	4	5	6	7	8	9	10	11	12	13	14	15	16	17	18	19	20	21	22	23	24	25
Cambozola & Smoked Ham Sandwich																									
Cheese & Celery Sandwich																									
Chicken Salad Sandwich																									
Chicken Tikka Sandwich																									
Chicken, Ham Mayonnaise & Lettuce Sandwich																									
Chicken, Smoked Ham & Mayonnaise Sandwich																									
Coronation Chicken Sandwich																									
Crunchy Cottage Cheese Sandwich																									
Egg Mayonnaise & Cress Sandwich																									
Egg, Bacon & Mayonnaise Sandwich																									
Egg, Mayonnaise & Bacon Roll																									
Garlic Sausage & Cream Cheese Sandwich																									

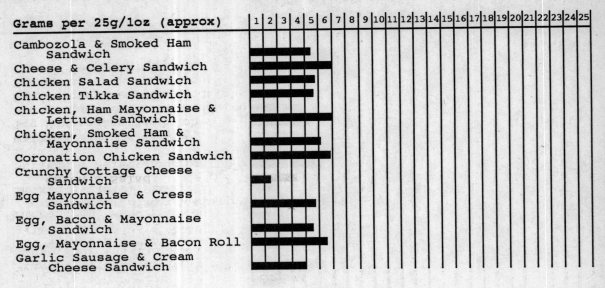

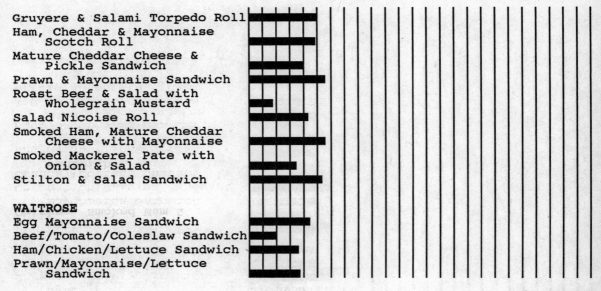

Gruyere & Salami Torpedo Roll

Ham, Cheddar & Mayonnaise
    Scotch Roll

Mature Cheddar Cheese &
    Pickle Sandwich

Prawn & Mayonnaise Sandwich

Roast Beef & Salad with
    Wholegrain Mustard

Salad Nicoise Roll

Smoked Ham, Mature Cheddar
    Cheese with Mayonnaise

Smoked Mackerel Pate with
    Onion & Salad

Stilton & Salad Sandwich

WAITROSE

Egg Mayonnaise Sandwich

Beef/Tomato/Coleslaw Sandwich

Ham/Chicken/Lettuce Sandwich

Prawn/Mayonnaise/Lettuce
    Sandwich

♦ = negligible

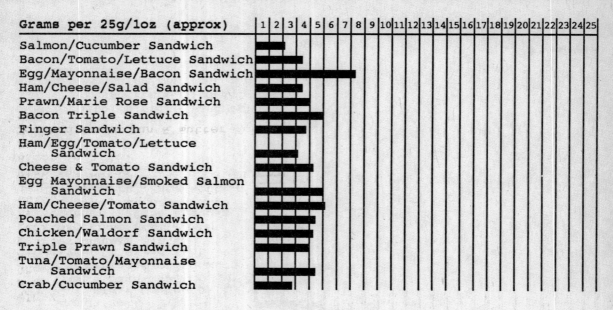

Grams per 25g/1oz (approx)	1	2	3	4	5	6	7	8	9	10	11	12	13	14	15	16	17	18	19	20	21	22	23	24	25
Salmon/Cucumber Sandwich																									
Bacon/Tomato/Lettuce Sandwich																									
Egg/Mayonnaise/Bacon Sandwich																									
Ham/Cheese/Salad Sandwich																									
Prawn/Marie Rose Sandwich																									
Bacon Triple Sandwich																									
Finger Sandwich																									
Ham/Egg/Tomato/Lettuce Sandwich																									
Cheese & Tomato Sandwich																									
Egg Mayonnaise/Smoked Salmon Sandwich																									
Ham/Cheese/Tomato Sandwich																									
Poached Salmon Sandwich																									
Chicken/Waldorf Sandwich																									
Triple Prawn Sandwich																									
Tuna/Tomato/Mayonnaise Sandwich																									
Crab/Cucumber Sandwich																									

Triple Filled Brioches

WIMPY
Hamburger
Cheeseburger
Kingsize
Quarterpounder
Quarterpounder with Cheese
Halfpounder
Chicken in a Bun
Spicy Beanburger with Cheese
Fish and Chips
Bacon in a Bun
Bacon/Egg in a Bun
Toasted Fruit Bun & Butter
Chips

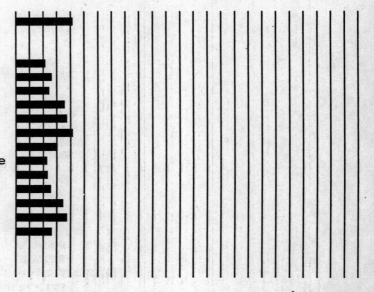

464

♦ = negligible